GW01316159

HOW T
TEACHING YOGA

10 steps to success

By Mark Bonington

Cover design by Samuel Hunt.
Model Suzanne Aitken.

www.markboningtonyoga.com

Note: Yoga and meditation are complimentary holistic practices intended to increase personal health and wellbeing. They are never to be used as a replacement for professional physical or mental help, or in place of medication.

Acknowledgements

For all the other aspiring yoga teachers.

This book would not have been possible without the brilliant team at Yoga London, with whom I undertook training in 2018.

Thank you also to the teams at MoreYoga, Virgin Active and Fitness First for trusting me to lead the weekly classes that I love!

To all my private clients: it's an honour to keep leading you through your yoga journeys.

Thank you to the beautiful Samuel Hunt for designing the beautiful covers.

And most especially, thank you to Suzanne Aitken, Lynn Bonington and John Bonington for their unsurpassed editing skills. Without their input, this guide would undoubtedly still be a messy draft on a hard drive.

CONTENTS

PREFACE: MY STORY

I remember very clearly the afternoon after I finished my yoga teacher training.

It had been the most incredible five weeks and I was fired up to start leading classes, my head still spinning from all that I had learned. But I remember two words, in particular, rattling around in my mind: "What now?"

What now?

Where to go from here?

Was it all a waste of time?

I had the certificate in my hand. I had the will and drive to teach my first yoga classes. I just had no idea how to take that first step. No, not a first step: the last step! The final step through the door and into the yoga studio, but this time on the other side of the mat – as the teacher.

Such a small step. Yet, in many ways, the most crucial one. The one that would make it all real and all happen.

But I had no idea how to make that transition; not a single clue as to how I was going to create those first opportunities. What follows in this guide will, I hope, help you on that journey. Maybe you are already a few steps ahead and have found your first classes. Maybe you are curious about how to transition from part-time to full-time teacher. Maybe you've not started your yoga teacher training yet and just want to look ahead for an idea of what happens after.

Maybe, like me in that summer of 2018, you are sitting on your bed with a certificate in your hand and many dreams of teaching yoga in your head, and not quite sure of how to make any of it happen.

Then this guide is, first and foremost, for you.

I'd like to start with a bit of background on how I found my-self sitting in my room, feeling more than a little apprehensive, with all the potential of being a great yoga teacher inside me but no idea as to how to make it manifest.

The truth is, I went to yoga teacher training because I didn't have anywhere else to go.

I had worked for several years in the intense world of digital marketing and corporate PR. A few months prior I had been offered a Director role in an agency, which I had thrown myself into, believing that it was the culmination of all my hard work and would propel me to new heights of success.

Half a year later I felt sick at the mere thought of going in to work. Every day was a department's worth of work on my shoulders and impossible deadlines with which to deliver it. Every hour was stress, anger, frustration, disappointment. Over and over and over. I didn't want to have anything to do with this job, this company, or this industry any more. I'd spent years doing this monotonous dance. I fought silently against it and yet the pressure to try and make it work invisibly bound me hour after hour, day after day, to a desk.

So I needed out.

I had no idea what I would do – I'd worked in media and marketing of some form or another for nigh-on seven years – but I screwed up my courage and handed in my notice. I finally started to accept that whatever the expectations of modern working were, I couldn't fulfil them; I couldn't button up my shirt and button up my opinions and click the day away. Whatever it took, whatever indeed it does take to do those jobs, I do not have it. Even if sometimes I wish that I did.

So I quit my PR job and, feeling like more or less an utter failure compared to everyone else I knew, decided to give a "real job" one last try by interviewing for a digital editor role at a travel magazine.

"And what will you do if you don't get the editor job?" my housemate at the time asked. I mentally scrabbled around for a plausible back-up plan that I did not have. "I will do my yoga teacher training," I replied, with more decisiveness than I felt.

Now, sure, I'd flirted in passing with the idea of becoming a yoga teacher in the three years that I'd been going to classes. I'd indulged it as a fantasy, even going so far as Googling courses in London and narrowing down my choices. I'd said to myself that this is what I'd do if all else failed, assuming that I'd never actually reach that point. Yet interestingly, that place we think of as rock-bottom can actually be rather liberating once you're there.

Well, all else certainly seemed to be failing fast, so I decided that if I wasn't successful in getting this journalism job then Yoga London and their one-month intensive could have me instead (though, obviously, I'd have to pay them to take me).

The agency I'd left asked if I could stay on as a part-time freelancer for a few months to lend my digital expertise to the team. Though reluctant, I agreed. At least I'd be guaranteed some sort of income whatever route things took, so I plugged away at the gruelling interview process for my newly desired digital editor role.

Well, one sunny Tuesday afternoon the email pinged into my inbox: while I had made it down to the final two, they had ultimately offered the role to the other candidate.

Fifteen minutes later I rang Yoga London. I explained that, having looked on their website, I could see that they had spaces on the course starting in two weeks. And while I understood candidates were supposed to have applied at least a couple of months in advance, they had space and I had a deposit. So could we make this work?

I was promptly fast-tracked through the application process and, two hours later, a much more welcome email popped into my inbox: I had secured my place on the one-month intensive 200-hour teacher training.

The course itself was a brilliant, enlightening, informative, sometimes frustrating but altogether treasured five weeks of my life. During the day my phone was off so I was untouchable by work emails, calls or social media. As London sweltered in a summer heatwave I learned about asanas, bandhas, chakras, koshas, doshas and anatomy. In the evenings and early mornings I drafted presentations, penned strategies and fired off emails in my new freelance role as a digital consultant.

And then, with a crash, the yoga course – my safe space when the rest of my world seemed entirely uncertain and altogether at sea – came to an end. Exams were passed, celebrations were had, drinks were shared and bonds of friendship were secured. But as it all started to fade there I was, sitting back on my bed. Alone, unsteady and unsure.

What now?

Little could I have known that six months later, at the opening of 2019, I would email that same agency, along with the other digital clients I had picked up along the way, to politely tell them that I was not looking for any more projects: from here on in I was a full-time yoga teacher.

It was a moment filled with liberation, a series of emails sent before I headed off to teach my Wednesday evening Hot Yoga class. It was the casting off of years of corporate frustration, the deep mental trauma of feeling trapped and acknowledging to myself that I had built a business which, while modest, allowed being a yogi to become my profession.

Here's the truth: it is possible. It's not always easy or straightforward and it's not always simple, but the things most worth devoting our time to rarely are. Whether you aspire to make a dramatic career change or use yoga to create a side-income, the opportunities are out there if you are prepared to look and go out of your way to make it happen.

Here's how to take yourself there.

Mark Bonington
London, August 2019

STEP 1: ASPIRATION & GETTING IT ALL IN ORDER

If you've recently finished your yoga teacher training, you probably have a million ideas on the go for your first classes. Maybe you've already started sequencing out your first flows, or thinking about the class themes, or working on meditation scripts.

All of that is great, and I would certainly encourage you to keep a notebook, journal or digital/app record of some kind to keep track of your ideas. But, the hard truth (and as you'll read, I'm all about hard truths when needed!) is that they will all mean nothing unless you can get yourself into a gym or studio to try them out. Let's get you there.

Now to be clear from the get-go, the techniques, tips and advice outlined in this guide are what worked for me as an aspiring yoga teacher in London, UK. But there is no reason that the principles and key takeaways could not apply anywhere where there is an appetite for yoga, an eager market for it and a teacher with some initiative. I am not an expert on sports/cultural law nor am I a financial advisor; I'm just someone who managed to make a living from yoga. So do always check any specific rules or laws around the teaching of yoga and setting yourself up as a fitness/wellbeing business wherever in the world you are.

First, sort your paperwork

Let's be honest: the paperwork bit is not glamorous and it's not fun, but if you have the important bits of paper to hand throughout your career as a yoga teacher, you will save yourself a lot of time and stress.

When you're starting out, this first and foremostly, includes three documents:

- Your training certificate
- Your insurance certificate
- Your CV

Have all of these sitting in their own folder, in PDF format, on your desktop. This is very important and we will come back to them later many times.

You may already be thinking that this sounds obvious as a first step, but I have spoken to plenty of new or aspiring yoga teachers who have yet to sort these all-important documents out.

Your yoga training certificate

I'm assuming your YTT school provided you with this. If possible, try to get them to send it to you a PDF copy along with a physical certificate. Many teachers take terrible, blurry pictures of their training certificate and try to send this when asked. The truth is this looks sloppy, unprofessional and wastes managers' time if they have to ask for a clearer image (which doesn't endear you to them – more on that later too).

If you have no choice but to take a picture on your phone, make sure it is high quality and the proportions are correct – basically the writing should be the right way round, I've been sent upside-down certificates in the past which I've had to personally edit. The same goes for any other certificates you plan on sending out, such as those for meditation or pregnancy yoga courses.

'Scannable' by Evernote is a handy little app that can help with this if you don't have your certificates on file as a PDF document, or aren't very good with image editing software.

Your training certificate is the proof that you have done the study and are ready to take a class, so put your best foot forward and make sure it's clear and easy to read – you're going to be asked for it a lot.

Yoga Insurance

Some yoga courses sort your first year of insurance out for you, so do check what comes with your teacher training package. Many, of course, do not and so you will need to fork out for this yourself.

Every gym or studio will ask for an insurance certificate, so if you want to teach professionally (even community or private classes) it is something you must have. Personally, I use DSC-Strand Ltd (Wellbeing Insurance). It costs about £50 a year and covers all forms of yoga and meditation teaching, including pregnancy and kids yoga. You can check them out at www.wellbeinginsurance.co.uk or drop a line to their customer service (which I found fast and helpful) at enquiries@wellbeinginsurance.co.uk.

A quick Google search will give you plenty of other options. Just make sure you've got your insurance certificate before proceeding as every venue you hope to teach at will ask you for it. It's a legal requirement.

Your Yoga CV

I imagine most readers will have created a CV of some sort before this, outlining things such as education, experience, personal information etc.

A yoga CV is similar but far more concise than a regular CV. Gyms and studios want to be able to see at no more than a single glance that you are properly qualified, have some experience and potentially have a bit of personality about you. Since you are not usually applying for salaried 'jobs' in the same way as a conventional recruitment process, I also opt for a picture on my CV so it's easy to identify after interviews or auditions.

Your yoga CV should be short, no more than a single page in length. And you can forget lists of hobbies and interests because none of that matters. All you need is your training (plus any additional workshops or masterclasses), the venues you've taught at, a few lines about you, the styles you are qualified in and comfortable to teach and any other relevant qualifications.

And while you want your CV to be easy on the eye it is much more important to make sure that it is easy to read. In an era when CV's seem to fast be becoming competitions in graphic design, less is most definitely more in the yoga world and you don't need to feel pressured to make it a work of art.

Here is mine for reference, almost one year to the day since I completed my teacher training:

MARK BONINGTON

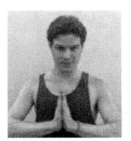

Address 17 XXX Street, London, W1X XXX

Telephone: +44 XXX XXX XXXX
Email: xxxxxxxxxxxxxx@gmail.com

Bringing a natural stage presence and theatricality to every class I teach, I have been practising yoga for over four years. I completed my RYT 200-hour with Yoga London in August 2018, specialising in Vinyasa Flow. Since then I have had the privilege to teach at gyms and studios across London in a variety of styles.

Highly motivated, I take great satisfaction in helping others find the inner and outer strength which yoga has taught me.

YOGA QUALIFICATIONS & FURTHER TRAINING

YOGA LONDON	**200-hour Yoga Alliance Certified**	**August 2018**
MoreYoga	**Yin + Meditation Masterclass**	**August 2019**
MoreYoga	**Dance Flow Workshop**	**July 2019**

YOGA TEACHING EXPERIENCE

Weekly Yoga Instructor   **MoreYoga, Fitness First, Virgin Active**   **Sept 2018 – Present**
The 52 Club

Leading weekly yoga and meditation classes, including Dynamic Vinyasa, Beginners and Hot Yoga, along with covering at various other branches across London.

Guided Meditation Teacher   **Urban Massage**   **Sept 2018 – Present**

Leading workshops and meditation sessions at corporate and public events, incorporating mindfulness, stress management and guided visualisation techniques.

Cover Yoga Instructor   **East of Eden, PureGym, Anytime Fitness,**   **August 2018 – Present**
AM Power Yoga, EnergyBase, H2 Clubs

Covering classes of various sizes, often at very short notice.

Private Yoga Instructor   **London-based Private Clients**   **August 2018 – Present**

Teaching one to one and in small groups, working with a variety of ability levels and injuries. Student goals were mainly improved strength, posture and flexibility, along with relaxation and mindfulness.

STYLES TAUGHT

Vinyasa Flow   Power Yoga   Hot Yoga   Yin   Meditation   Ashtanga   Hatha   Restorative

---

ADDITIONAL SKILLS

- Published journalist, writer and copywriter
- Digital marketer and social media expert
- Trained singer and actor

OTHER EDUCATION

University of Dundee   **English Literature (2:1)**   **July 2010**

Why become a yoga teacher?

If you're taking a break editing your CV together or waiting for replies to emails as you sort out the above, now is the perfect time to set out your reasons for becoming a yoga teacher. After all, there are many things you could have invested time and money into in order to generate a new stream of income, so why yoga?

Start with why. This comes from a now-(in)famous phrase coined by Simon Sinek in his popular TED Talk. But starting with the 'why' of why you want to teach yoga can be a powerful way to connect with what your goals are as you step into the realms of professional teaching.

Perhaps you want to do something where you're helping people or which offers you the chance to give back to your community?

Could it be that you want a side income from something which indulges your love of the spiritual practices?

Perhaps you're simply sick of sitting at a desk all day?

Whatever your reasons are, take some time to consider them and write them down. Be completely honest. You don't have to show them to anyone else; these are just a touchstone for your teaching and they will be invaluable down the line when you start to question what you're doing and why you're doing it.

It could be that you've already considered these – in my own yoga teacher training sharing a reason why we'd chosen to invest time in becoming a teacher was one of the first group ice-breaker exercises. If so, remember them and write them down.

Relating it back to my own story, my 'why' was:

- **Genuineness:** Working in PR/marketing had made me very good at manipulation: Manipulation of clients, of customers and of viewers/readers. I was sick of it and wanted something which I felt offered a more genuine face-to-face human interaction.

- **Less screen time:** I'd had side-hustles before, but they'd always just involved more time sitting in from of various screens. I wanted to earn extra income by doing something dynamic and physical.

- **Simplicity:** There is a clarity in offering a set service for a set amount of time. I was bored by the corporate world blurring the lines between work-time and free-time with incessant "company culture" outings and wanted those lines more definitively drawn.

Journaling your yoga journey

Keeping a yoga journal is an excellent way of tracking your learnings as a yoga teacher and I would highly recommend starting one, even if you're not a journaler already. Like other aspects outlined above this may have already been a key part of your YTT, if so it's simply a case of carrying it on.

Personally, I find writing longhand on pen and paper the best and most freeing way to keep a yoga journal, but I also have documents filed on places like Google Drive and the Notebook app. The beauty of journaling is that there are no rules, so go with the medium and style which best suits your personality.

If the concept of keeping a journal is new to you, then what better starting point than your aspirations as a yoga teacher?

Other ideas to track in your yoga journal include:

- Themes for classes or personal practice
- Peak postures and the flows to get there
- Quotes from teachers/anyone who inspire you
- Ideas for intentions (both for class and your personal practice)
- Asanas/postures you find particularly difficult and your progress on them

- Meditation diary
- Studies into yoga history/philosophy you've under-taken
- Anatomical and alignment cues to use in class
- Anything else which takes your fancy!

Keeping a yoga journal allows you to track where your teaching journey began and, over time, how it has evolved. It can be extremely satisfying to look back and see how far you have come over the weeks and months. At the same time, sometimes you need to look back and remember why you began this journey in the first place.

Setting goals

Now that you have a better idea of why you want to teach yoga, spend some time setting out your short and long-term goals of what you want to achieve.

How you go about this will very much depend on who you are as a person and how you operate. It could be that you have a set amount of income you want to make per week/per month with yoga teaching (in which case my advice would be to make sure it's realistic, as the average pay for an hour's class in London is £30).

Or it could be that you have set your sights on a particular gym or studio you'd like to work for. Again, keep a sense of realism here. As a new (or relatively new) teacher in a highly competitive market, the premier yoga outlets are not likely to be interested until you have a bit of experience under your belt.

In terms of timeframe this can vary from venue to venue (some are happy to take teachers fresh from training), but other gyms/studios will want a minimum of one year's experience, while others may demand as many as three to five years or more.

Short-term goals
Consider where you want to be in the next 3-6 months. Take into account how much time you will have to devote to teaching yoga

and what you will need to prepare in order to take you there (including the essential documents outlined previously).

Potential short-term goals include:

- Securing your first cover classes
- Growing your network with new yoga teachers and gym managers
- Successfully joining online cover groups
- Landing your first permanent weekly class
- Landing your first private client

Long-term goals
Consider where you want to be in the next 6-12 months and beyond. What are the fundamental steps you want to be on your way to achieving when it comes to your yoga teaching career? These will likely need to be broken down further with month-to-month steps and short-term goals as they will take a longer period to come to fruition.

Potential long-term goals could include:

- Building a weekly timetable of several public classes in gyms/studios
- Creating your own community classes
- Building a roster of private clients
- Opening your own studio
- Moving your yoga teaching from a part-time to full-time occupation

So set our your goals, keeping them personal to you and you alone, and then file them in your yoga journal.

Managing expectations

The purpose of this guide is in no way, at any point, to rain on anyone's parade. I encourage every yoga teacher, at whatever level they find themselves, to dream on and dream big. Yoga isn't going anywhere and the more yoga teachers there are the more yoga there is. And that can only be a good thing given the state of the world right now.

Yet it has been my experience, both as a relatively recent graduate and from observing yogis fresh from training who have come after me, that there can be some unrealistic expectations flying around as to what is possible, at least in the first instance, when it comes to making use of your teaching diploma.

We will dive more deeply into cultivating the right attitude in Chapter 4, but to begin simply finding gratitude for what you can get is the best place you can start. If you think that a week out of your training you'll be teaching your very own Vinyasa Flow class at TriYoga, you're going to be disappointed. I've seen new yoga teachers turn their nose up at teaching opportunities at discount gyms, community spaces or even classes aimed at beginners. As you'll see, every chance to teach is a chance to grow your skills, make new connections and forge new opportunities.

The truth is that, when you start out, you're not above anything except teaching for free (never let yourself be talked into this unless it's for charity). And as mentioned, premium yoga brands can demand up to five years of experience before they will even consider an application from you. Not to mention that above your basic training some will even demand specialisation training in a particular style, such as Rocket or Yin, or that you have gone through their particular teacher training school.

There is nothing wrong with aspiring to a particular name, but temper those eager expectations; accept that many of the teachers who stand in those institutions have worked hard for years to be there. As a tadpole in the pond, one day you can be there too, but you have to be methodical in your approach. To borrow an appropriate quote from Dwayne Johnson: "Success isn't always about greatness. It's about consistency. Consistent hard work leads to success."

If you keep an open mind as to the opportunities which come

your way, then there's no reason you can't start down that Yellow Brick Road straight away and lay the foundations that lead to your dream yoga job.

STEP 2: FIND YOUR
FIRST COVER CLASSES

So, with our essential documents in hand, goals set and expectations managed, what's the next step?

Your way into yoga teaching is usually by covering other teachers. In this chapter, I will outline some of the ways you can find your first classes, before exploring how to use each one to create more opportunities for yourself in the subsequent chapter. I strongly suggest you read and absorb both together as they are very much two sides of the same coin when it comes to those all-important first steps.

Personal contacts

I was very envious of fellow trainees who had access to this one when going through the teacher training as, coming from the corporate world, I had no experience whatsoever in the worlds of fitness or wellness. And no experience meant no contacts. Or so I thought.

Naturally, if you are already working in a gym or studio in some capacity, use anyone you know. If you're already teaching in another form, such as PT or dance, get the emails of any Group Exercise Managers (GXIs) that you can and get emailing with those CVs, insurance and certs.

As I racked my brains following the end of my training, the only light I could come up with was the gym where I had done the majority of my classes. After enquiring at reception, and doing a little digging with the other teachers, I had the name of the right head office contact to email and get on the audition list. It was a start.

Also remember that your fellow trainees are all potential contacts within the industry now, too. In the weeks following the end of your training, consider roping everyone's numbers together in a WhatsApp group and sharing any cover opportunities which you can't do. Be each other's support rather than each other's rivals and see what comes of it.

Keep in mind always that, even in our interconnected digital age, word of mouth and personal recommendation is the most powerful form of marketing that there is. Much more on this to come!

Facebook cover groups

This was without a doubt my #1 way of getting my foot through a number of different yoga teaching doors.

Facebook has many closed cover groups especially for yoga and they can be an invaluable tool when it comes to getting started if you search them out. My recommendations for groups at this writing are:

- Yoga and Pilates Cover Teachers London
- Yoga Instructors London – Cover Group
- Cover me Yoga UK

Obviously these are primarily geared towards London/UK, but you get the general idea. There are many variations and regional groups out there designed to connect yoga teachers in a particular geographic area. Have a search through Facebook and see what you find.

Play by the rules

Most of these groups are private and you will need to fill out a form in order to join. The admins will want proof that you are a genuine yoga teacher looking for cover opportunities before they approve you – some will even want to see a copy of those documents from Chapter 1 (starting to see why they're so important yet?).

Fill out the answers as honestly and succinctly as you can and be patient when waiting for approval to join. It can sometimes take a few days.

When you are approved, make sure you give the group rules a read (some groups pin this as a post to the top of the page). These rules are strict and violating them is a one-way ticket to being banned, which is the last thing you want, particularly at this stage. Yoga cover groups are understandably insistent that all posts are cover-related to keep the content as relevant as possible, so avoid posting personal marketing or life updates. Even "Hi! I'm a new teacher looking for opportunities..." may not be allowed.

And to be honest, such a generic plea for work probably isn't going to get you anything.

The need for speed

Here's an insider secret that I learned fast: Cover opportunities do not go to the most qualified or experienced teacher. Usually they go to the yogi who replies quickest!

In a competitive yoga market such as London, you usually have only a few minutes, at most, to nab a new opportunity before it's snatched by someone else. So how can you speed up the process?

Here are some top tips from my own experience:

1. Make sure your phone settings allow Facebook updates to appear on your home/locked screen so you can see the moment someone in the cover group posts an opportunity. You can adjust these in your phone settings under the options for the Facebook App.

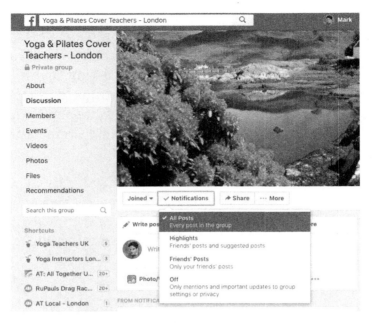

2. Make sure your Facebook settings are configured to update you about every post to the group – often by default you will only see "highlights". To ensure you are kept up to date, go to the cover group page, click on 'Notifications' at the top and make sure 'All Posts' is selected (see image above).

3. That fast-access folder on your desktop with your yoga CV and certs in it. This will save you precious seconds when applying for cover as there will be no need to rifle through your documents and files looking for them – you can promptly drag and drop.

4. When a cover opportunity comes up that you can do, comment underneath immediately (why hesitate?), tagging the @name of the poster if possible and informing them that you can take it. Immediately send them a private message (PM) on Facebook too, dragging and dropping your CV/certs into the message and including a line or two about your training/experience so far.

Follow the above guidelines and it won't be long until you've landed your first cover opportunity.

No experience yet? No problem

Everybody starts somewhere. If you're shy on experience then play up your training. If you took a turn teaching the class during your training, then you were a "teaching assistant" at one point. If you taught friends one to one or in small groups to practice, then you've had private clients and classes. The fact they perhaps paid you in Deliveroo and gratitude rather than cash is neither here nor there at this point.

For obvious reasons you can't overtly lie on your CV and pretend that you've had experience when you haven't, and it would be very foolish to try, but you can put your best foot forward and show your eagerness to progress in your teaching while milking the experience you've already acquired.

"Payroll only"

As you see cover opportunities come through, some may come with the addendum "Payroll only". For brands such as Virgin Active, Fitness First, GymBox and others, you have to already be on their payment system to cover a class. Many yoga studios operate on this basis too.

It can quickly start to sound like a frustrating catch-22; you can't cover unless you've already covered before or have gone through their audition process.

But here's an insider secret: when it comes down to the 11th hour, gyms and studios will do anything not to have to cancel the class on their members, so if there are only a few hours to go it can still be worth pitching yourself to the "payroll only" opportunities, particularly if you already have some cover experience under your belt or live close to the venue.

We will discuss auditions more in-depth in Chapter 5, but if you are keen to audition for branded gyms and studios most will have information on their website on how to get in contact. If not, dropping the brand a line on Facebook messenger is a good way to find more information.

Don't waste anyone's time

Most importantly, your own. It can feel tempting when looking for your first covers to apply for anything and everything. But be realistic. Choose classes you will feel relatively comfortable teaching (keeping in mind that everyone gets nervous) and that are worth your time to travel to. For cover, teachers want some assurance that you are going to be able to turn up on time and confidently step into the breach.

Bear in mind that if a cover class is in an unfamiliar style or miles away from where you live, cultivating a relationship with that studio is not going to serve you long-term. And as we will soon see, even with one-off cover work you should always be looking at the bigger picture.

Final word on finding cover

Anyone who knows me knows that I am not a patient person; when I want something I tend to go after it heart and soul. But patience is indeed a virtue when it comes to landing those first cover classes.

Remember that as a teacher fresh from training, you are starting at the bottom of the heap. And in major cities such as London the heap of yoga teachers is large and growing by the day. That said, there are new gyms and studios opening all the time, businesses looking to offer yogic practices to their employees and communities crying out for their own yoga classes.

You will have to sell yourself hard, especially at the start, and be open to classes not in your immediate area (though again, keep it realistic). My philosophy to begin was that, if it was accessible by Tube, under an hour of travel and fairly paid, I would take it. So after only a few weeks my CV was looking a lot healthier.

Stay persistent and it will not be long before you land your first class.

STEP 3: YOUR CLASS PREPARATIONS

OK, so let's assume you've successfully pitched and won your first cover class. Chances are you're feeling pretty nervous, right? Don't worry, you're not alone. Before my first 30-strong cover class at PureGym I felt like I was about to be asked to step onto a stage and improvise an entire opera single-handed.

Nerves are normal, especially when you're covering. I can say now from experience it is much less intimidating going into a weekly class which you've been given than covering someone else's.

Why? Well because, first and foremost, the members were likely expecting the listed teacher. Many yogis get attached less to a particular style and more to an individual teacher (think back to your own experiences as a yoga practitioner for the truth of this). So when they've fallen sick or gone off on holiday, students are not always as thrilled as we'd like to see a cover teacher step to the front of the class. That's the hard truth.

Your challenge as a cover teacher, therefore, is to rise up and prove your right to lead those students. Here's how to give yourself the best chance possible to do that and set yourself up for good things to follow.

Arrive early

One of the best ways to calm your own nerves is to arrive at the venue in plenty of time. My standard, especially if the location is unfamiliar, is at least 15-20 minutes before the designated start time. That might seem excessive but here's why:

- **5-10 minutes** to account for travel delays or unforeseen circumstances. They will arise when you least want them.

- **5 minutes** to get changed (if needed) and find the appointed room. Some gyms, especially in cities, are now vast sprawling labyrinths comprising scores of halls and studios. Finding your way around in an unfamiliar venue can be a time-consuming challenge.

- **5 minutes** to get the music set up and (silently) swear at the sound system as you twiddle with the dials in an attempt to get the overhead speakers to play.

Oh yes, you'll have great fun with some of those sound systems. I certainly have. Don't worry, you soon figure them out. If not, ask the person at reception for help – they usually take sympathy if you're covering and unfamiliar with the in-house tech.

Presentation is everything

My Dad has a great phrase about this which I've always remembered: "You only get one chance at a first impression".

And when you're a working cover yoga teacher, you want to make a lasting impression on those members. Get them on side and the opportunities are far more likely to follow (more on that later).

I've spoken to yoga teachers who quite happily slob out of bed, throw on the previous day's gym kit and roll on into their first class.

Now granted, we've all had days like that. But when you're covering, you want to come to class looking like you mean business (even if that business is teaching yoga). This is a personal teaching philosophy I've carried forward since the start of my yoga career.

Maybe it's my corporate client-facing background, maybe it's just me. I'm not sure.

But either way, I'm 100% sure that when I arrive early, freshly showered and with clean kit on, I feel far more confident about stepping to the front of a class to lead it. It also does a lot to soothe my nerves if it's a class I'm unfamiliar with or feel nervous about leading.

Yes, I do still get nervous even after more than a year of teaching yoga. It's still a challenge, albeit a wonderfully welcome one, and just like any good performance sometimes those nerves help to push me even further.

The cover teacher philosophy

No doubt as a new teacher you already have a boatload of ideas for how you want to structure classes, maybe ways that you want to style your teaching or physical/spiritual sources of inspiration to draw from. Keep writing them down in your yoga journal so that you can refer back and develop them as your teaching career progresses. They're incredibly useful on the days or times when the mind decides to draw a blank.

But hard truth time again: cover classes are not the place to be wildly experimental.

Stay true to your personal style as a teacher, but keep in mind that your job as a cover teacher is to give the class what they were already expecting, insomuch as you can. You want the flows to reflect this, usually being open-level (accessible to all practitioners, unless the class description specifically states otherwise), incorporating standard yoga asanas/poses and following classic class structure.

For guidance, I would outline a 'classic' yoga class structure as follows:

- Opening meditation/intention-setting and warm-up

- Heat-building flow sequences (sun salutes or equivalent), leading into:
- Standing/balance sequences
- Seated/deep stretch or strength sequences
- Cool down/relaxation sequence

A good starting point when designing your first cover class is to look up the class title on the gym/studio website and see how they describe it. Go with that description, being aware that you may need to speed up or slow down the pace of the class on-the-fly if the practitioner level is higher or lower than you initially predicted.

While I don't want to put any dampeners on your creativity or discourage you from bringing your unique personality into the room, I know from experience that the best way to success as a cover teacher is to keep the yoga class very standard.

Your essential yoga teaching toolkit

With your class plan on hand and hopefully in your head, there are a few key essentials to have on your person when you're travelling around teaching yoga.

- **Smartphone or Tablet (with any adaptors needed)**. Personally, I found a tablet to be a great investment as a yoga teacher, as it meant that I could fill a room with just my device if need be. Full overhead sound systems are always preferable, but the threat of technical difficulties is always there and knowing I can crank up the volume on my iPad is a great comfort.

If, like me, you're also an Apple user, then make sure you have your own adaptor handy as they (oh-so-helpfully) no longer make headphone jacks on their products. Gyms and studios do not always provide these (or if they do they're "borrowed" on a weekly basis) and most sound systems still use a standard headphone jack attachment.

- **Aux cable.** This is the attachment that goes from your smart device into the sound system. Again, the gym or studio should provide this but many do not, so always best to have one on you. You can buy aux cables pretty cheaply from Amazon or any electronics shop.

- **Music playlist.** Have your playlists downloaded and able to play offline as WiFi connection is not guaranteed in many venues (or if it is, with so many users online, it can be a dodgy connection at best). Keep in mind that you cannot play music if the venue does not hold a license, which is always worth checking. These are expensive so some venues ask that you use their own pre-made playlists or SoundCloud tracks, or even royalty-free public domain music, so it's always worth checking what the policy on playing music is.

More info on music and designing your own class playlists can be found below.

- **Change of kit**. If you end up getting soaked, sitting on something nasty or spilling your lunch down yourself on the way over a change of kit is an incredible relief. Always carry one with you.

- **Water.** Essential, always.

Notes on music

Music can be one of the most fun, interesting and creative ways to theme and individualise your classes. It is a wonderful way to add to the atmosphere you are trying to create in the space and compliment the themes you are weaving with your sequences, whether this is the fiery high-intensity of a Power Flow class or prompting the inner reflection and deep relaxation of a Restorative class.

Yet initially, to be entirely honest, I didn't spend a great deal of time putting playlists together; I simply added a collection of ambient tracks together from which I could hit 'shuffle' and get on with the teaching.

As time has gone on, I've taken the mixing more seriously and have a clearer idea of how I want the structure of the music to match the structure of the class. Putting the playlists together is now a key part of my week and one of the ways I try to bring some personality into my yoga classes. As you can see from my Spotify (link below) I also love experimenting with themes and styles when it comes to ordering the tracks.

While much of the music contains the cool, meditative vibes and eastern-style influences you would expect from a yoga class, I also draw inspiration from everything from contemporary pop music to film and video game scores.

Music licensing

I'm no expert when it comes to licensing law but, as mentioned above, it is always worth checking if you are allowed to play music in the venue in which you are teaching. Most major gyms/studios have commercial music licenses, but not all and if you are looking at setting up your own public classes you will need one of your own.

This is simply one of those areas in which you do not want to be caught out and slapped with a nasty fine, so always play by the rules, read up and double-check.

Playlist structure

When I design class playlists, I try to open with gentle tracks to ease the class into the meditation and warm-up, before picking up the beat for sun salutes/flows/standing and strength sequences, then slowing it down with meditative beats for deep stretches and savasana.

For a Power/Vinyasa class, the music stays upbeat for longer as the class has a higher energy. For a Hatha/Gentle class the music stays more subdued to mirror the periods for inner reflection in the class as poses are held for longer, and in my Yin playlists there are not any upbeat tracks whatsoever.

I sometimes incorporate pop tracks by artists like Madonna (Ray of Light is a gorgeous album to lift yoga music from), Britney or Paloma Faith, but in general these are few and far between. Even lighter pop songs have lyrics deliberately designed to grab and hold the attention, which isn't what you want when trying to create a reflective atmosphere, so use them sparingly. The most important aspect of a good playlist is that the tracks flow seamlessly into one another and become pleasant background noise, not the main focus of the class.

The more you teach the more you will come to understand how you like to structure your classes, and the music will naturally become an aspect of this. One hot tip is not to open the playlist with the track you want to use – have 5-10 minutes of 'background' music first to give yourself and the students time to arrange themselves, grab blocks etc and do your opening class checks.

If you're unsure how to make your own yoga playlists for now, my own are public and available on Spotify. If you want to check them out or use them you can find me under username "mbono", searching "Mark Bonington" or following this link (https:// open.spotify.com/user/mbono).

No music?

Some yoga teachers deliberately keep musical input into classes to a minimum, or do not use it at all, as it can be another distraction which takes students out of their internally-focused practise and concentration on the body and breath.

How much you use music is, of course, up to you and will reflect your individual style of teaching, but not using any is a perfectly valid option (and some venues have this as their house policy).

Summary on cover classes

Cover classes are likely to be where you start as a yoga teacher, and I've seen several yoga teachers in my time, even ones fresh from graduation, who have turned their nose up at cover opportunities because they were not in their immediate area, not in a top-notch/branded venue or didn't feel the pay was high enough.

While you have to set yourself a value of what you know you are worth as a yoga teacher, you also have to accept your place in the market and take the work which comes your way, especially at the start. Keep in mind that every single cover opportunity is a chance to sow the seeds of future success.

I experienced all of the above frustrations when starting out as my first few months as a yoga teacher consisted primarily of covering. But with patience and persistence those early covers led to weekly classes on the timetable, which led to work in other venues and private clients.

I have found that the difference between success and failure in this is largely down to two things: being consistent with the work and cultivating the right attitude, which we will explore next.

STEP 4: ATTITUDE

Success in all those previous steps relies on one thing: attitude.

If you step into those first classes with the mindset of an entrepreneur creating a one-man/one-woman business you will find far more success than if you think of yourself as simply a yoga teacher looking for gigs in a crowded market. This applies whether your aspiration is a dramatic change of career or simply turning a beloved hobby into a side stream of income.

And you never know, one may lead to the other. It did for me.

First, you're not above anything

I've mentioned this before, but this is one I have encountered repeatedly from yoga teachers, especially if they are new. There truly is an idea sometimes that, once the teacher training course is over, the hard work is done and a new teacher can sit at home and wait to be called by a top studio.

Nope. Doesn't work like that. If you want to make it happen, you have to go out and make it so. The true hard work starts after your final exams end.

Your initial cover work will probably not be in the most glamorous spots, with students who do not have the most advanced practice (which limits how creative and dynamic you can be with those flows), for not a great amount of money.

So a key part of yoga success at the start is adopting the right attitude: Find an enjoyment in those first classes and accept that nobody owes you anything. See each one as a step in your yoga teaching career and resolve to make the most out of every one that you can.

As stated, unless it's Karma Yoga or charity/community classes, the only thing you are above is working for free.

The entrepreneur mindset

Shift your thinking from "I'm a yoga teacher" to "I run my own yoga business" right from the start.

The difference may be subtle, but the attitude that comes from an open vs a closed mindset is, I have found, vastly different. An entrepreneur explores every opportunity to sell their product/service to new clients and is constantly looking to tap into sources and markets that may have been overlooked by their peers.

The entrepreneur sees it as a challenge to stand out and make their mark on a particular industry, even when it is already crowded. This mindset is creative and always looking for new outlets, even in unexpected corners (sometimes especially in those areas!), whereas boxing yourself into the "yoga teacher" stereotype limits you to try and do simply what all the other yoga teachers are doing.

In the case of contemporary yoga, as you will no doubt have seen, this entrepreneurial mindset has spawned the creation of several sub-industries to cater to different parts of the market as it grows. This ranges from classes aimed at different ages or genders, to creating compliments to other spiritual practices, to yoga involving anything from alcohol to animals.

This is why starting with your goals and reasons for teaching yoga is both powerful and important – if you feel disheartened (and any entrepreneur's journey is going to involve a certain amount of rejection and heartache) go back to those core reasons of why you started teaching and reconnect with them.

Down the line, that kernel and key question of "why" may even encourage you to find your preferred niche within the yoga market, or perhaps even create one of your own.

Make every cover class count

So, you may have already applied what is in the previous chapters and begun landing your first cover classes. Well done! Taking the initiative is very much a key part of cultivating the right attitude.

Yet as the initial thrill of teaching starts to wear off it's very easy to become disheartened at the start of your yoga career. Let's be realistic: one-off classes for £30 (or less in some cases) don't feel like much. As previously mentioned, I felt stuck in this space for the first couple of months of my teaching career at least. I was covering a lot, but it was frustrating not to see all that cover work lead to more.

I discovered it was paramount to look beyond the individual fee of each cover class and see every single one as a gateway opportunity for future work.

Let's look at what this means in more detail:

1. **Get the students on your side**

Give the best class you can give, always remembering that you are there to provide a service to the students and their practice, not your own. Too many teachers see teaching yoga as an extension of their own practice when truthfully it's the opposite – you're there to aid the practice of others.

At the end of your cover class, humbly ask the members to leave a review or let the management know if they enjoyed your class. Most gyms/studios have a system for this, whether it is via their booking app, written feedback cards or on the website.

Managers are constantly monitoring these feedback streams as part of their job; which is, first and foremost, is to keep their members happy. If they see your name repeatedly coming up in positive reviews, it dramatically increases the chances they will keep you in mind for future class covers or permanent classes on the timetable.

The students need to be your cheerleaders as they are the most important asset and life-blood for any gym or studio. Get them on side and you're onto a winner.

2. **Get the management to follow**

The way you endear yourself to the management is slightly different. Essentially, make their job as easy as possible. File your invoices for any cover classes on time and in the venue's preferred format. Read payment procedures carefully (some involve several steps and multiple emails) and follow them to the letter.

Many yoga teachers neglect this side and repeatedly do not pay attention to the individual admin procedures of different gyms, or even expect the venue to cater to them, which wastes management's time with chasing and follow-up.

Make the manager's job easy as a freelancer and you will stand out from the crowd.

3. **Arm yourself with business cards and sell yourself**

This is another hangover I took from the corporate world. It's something that many yoga teachers do not bother with, but which can be an invaluable tool for generating new business.

Think of every student in every class you teach as a potential new private client. Now, granted, most will not have the time or money for private yoga lessons, but some will. I have generated new regular private clients off the back of classes in discount gyms or one-off covers, and a large part of this was having a business card to give to the student for them to follow up with.

After every class, make your sales pitch: Invite students to take one of your cards with them and stay in touch, follow you on Instagram, or keep you in mind if they are interested in one to one yoga. Keep in mind that as soon as a class ends some students will be putting their mat away and heading out the door, so you only have a single line or two at most to sell yourself and your services.

4. Take the initiative and follow up

Even with all of the above, there are a lot (and growing) number of yoga teachers also looking for those same opportunities. Yet in any form of business it always surprised me how often, in our technologically connected world, people would not take the initiative. Even when it was as simple as sending an email.

When the final 'Om' has been chanted and the final mantra closed on your cover class, the work is not over. Follow up with the manager or teacher you covered for and thank them for the opportunity. Mention that you enjoyed it, had great feedback from the students, and would be interested in any further opportunities in future. You just never know what's coming – they may be going on holiday next month, or they might have a timetable clash the very next week.

If you are known as a reliable and organised teacher, you will be front of mind for future cover work or even permanent weekly classes down the line.

Rejection

As mentioned previously, rejection is part of any entrepreneur's journey. When we are building something for ourselves, especially when that something is reliant on our own services and skill set, it can deepen the sting of the rejection significantly.

Why? Because it can feel like it is not just our ideas or work that is being rejected but our individual person too.

Let's be real: Rejection is never fun nor is it usually what we would choose for ourselves. But we can choose how we handle it and the lessons we draw from it.

Rejection by gyms or studios

This can come in a number of forms, perhaps a cover at a particular place that never resulted in anything further (as I said, I had plenty), perhaps an audition that didn't go the way you hoped (more on auditions in the next chapter).

Sometimes the truth is that, no matter how many of the boxes you tick, some opportunities do not manifest into more. At least not in the immediate, even if the feedback was great and you followed all of the above. But remember that "no" sometimes just means "not yet". And keep in mind that sometimes it's a slow-burn and you may not hear anything for several weeks or even months.

How you teach is directly tied to your personality and, unfortunately, you will not be a fit for every opportunity that comes your way. Studios, especially, often like to teach in a particular style (some even have set sequences their teachers must adhere to), and they need to know that all individuals on their books are a match for what the clientele will be expecting. More often than not, when it doesn't lead to more, it's because of them, not because of you.

Take all you can from the experience and apply it to your next opportunities.

Rejection from individuals

In the same way that not every gym or studio will be a fit for you professionally, not every student is going to enjoy your classes. Again, simply fact. You cannot please everyone no matter how middle of the road you go.

For most, this will simply mean that they do your class and leave, and should you appear on the timetable in future they will opt to go to other classes. Some students, however, will feel the need to tell you precisely why they did not enjoy your class. Sometimes this is constructive feedback and should be welcomed, sometimes it can veer into something more aggressive.

Particularly when covering, some students (somehow) expect you to teach *exactly* like the teacher you are covering for and even mimic their sequences. While you do want to stick to the style outlined in the class description, as mentioned before, it's impossible to truly imitate another teacher and unwise to try.

I have experienced this first hand, where not only did a student try to interrupt my class to tell me I was doing it all wrong, they accosted me afterwards to tell me I clearly knew nothing about yoga, that I was not a patch on the previous teacher who taught the class and I had no teaching talent whatsoever.

I'm grateful that this experience did not happen within my first week of teaching and covering my first classes, but I can't say that it didn't affect me. Thankfully, many other people have given me great feedback, before and since (including other students from that same class), and those are the comments to remember when someone tries to bring you down.

I can't say I understand why people think they have the right to throw their criticism at someone who is simply trying to provide the best teaching service possible, but it is more a reflection on them and their own issues than it is you and your teaching prowess.

Rejection hurts, but put on as positive an attitude as you can and move on.

Imposter Syndrome

This occurs in all sorts of professions and at every level. Essentially imposter syndrome is that little voice saying that you don't deserve to be where you are; that there is someone who can do it better than you or deserves to be there more than you do. Many of those who suffer with imposter syndrome also speak of a fear of being "found out" or "revealed as a fraud" and the anxiety around losing everything they have built.

It's entirely normal to feel this way. We all have those little inner demon voices which nibble away at our confidence and niggle us throughout the day. Some of the biggest talents in the world, from technical entrepreneurs to opera superstars, have spoken about how they battle with feeling like a fraud when standing up in front of a crowd.

The cure for imposter syndrome is, first and foremost, to remind yourself that you do deserve to be there at the front of the room. You've done the training, you've made the opportunity, and you have every right to stand in front of that class and teach them yoga.

Secondly, the best way I've found to silence those voices is to do the work beforehand – if I've prepared my class plan, arrived on time and done all I can to give the attendees the best class possible, then there's little I can reprimand myself with even if something goes wrong or someone clearly didn't chime with my teaching.

Remember also that little mistakes and flaws are just part of being human. You're a living, breathing teacher, not a machine. All yoga teachers occasionally stumble in a sequence or forget to do a pose on the left that they did on the right. The truth is that most of the time the students will be too focused on their own practice to even notice. And even if they do, the world will keep on turning.

When it comes down to it, if you don't have confidence in your own abilities as a teacher, how can you expect anyone else to?

Positive mental attitude

As you start to amass positive feedback from your classes, it can be beneficial to note these in your yoga journal. On days when you feel it's not going as well as you hoped, it can be incredibly affirming to look back and remember.

Sometimes, as yoga teachers, it seems like we are somehow expected to be immune from such mundane, everyday things as hurt or criticism, jealousy or fear; as though once we are handed our teaching certificate we are magically granted enlightenment and freed from mortal sufferings. I can't speak for anyone else, but most of the yoga teachers I know are still wonderfully human!

We all have days when we don't feel like we're worth it, when we feel burned out or as though we are not good enough. But part of fostering the right attitude is finding the positive even when things do not go precisely the way you would have liked. Keeping a note of your wins can be incredibly helpful and comforting during such times, when you can look back and see how far you've grown as a teacher, and as a person.

From attitude to opportunity

Another great way to weather professional rejection, imposter syndrome or any opportunities that did not go the way you hoped is to have multiple projects on the go at once. This way if one falls by the wayside it does not feel like your entire yoga teaching career is going up in smoke.

As we've explored part of the entrepreneurial mindset and cultivating the right attitude is not focusing all the energy in one place but applying your talents, in this case your top-notch yoga teaching skills, anywhere and everywhere that you can.

And one of the gateways that every aspiring yoga teacher must go through at some point when chasing those new opportunities is auditions.

STEP 5: AUDITIONS

Sometimes covering classes in a venue, and getting good feedback on them from members, will grant you something of a "pass" onto the cover list and payment system. For other places, they will want you to audition before you're even allowed to cover a class.

Auditions are something that every modern yoga teacher will encounter at some point. They can be nerve-wracking, in particular because it can be hard to gauge what a particular gym or studio is looking for, and to know what you should prepare.

Sadly, auditions are by no means passable with a "one size fits all" attitude, but I will try to outline here the main points and learnings I have found from attending various auditions, some of which I passed and some of which I did not.

But I can say that every single one was a steep learning curve.

Landing auditions

Auditions are anomalies and can really come from anywhere and everywhere. Sometimes new studios, or established chains looking to grow their roster of teachers, will post open auditions on those Facebook cover groups we explored in Chapter 2. Another great reason to be on them and check updates regularly.

When you go through a gym or studio's official website, following your online application, they may book you in for an audition. Or you could be referred by a friend or colleague; many paths lead to the audition room. Once you're in there, you'll have only a few vital minutes to show what you can do.

Research

Just as with many other aspects of building a yoga career, research is key. Long before you set foot in the audition room it is a powerful place to begin. What does a studio's website, the current roster of teachers and social media presence tell you about them?

The devil is often in the details here, so look closely. If they often make humorous or light-hearted quips, then you may want to reflect this in your audition script. Look to see how much Sanskrit they use when describing poses – some studios like to embrace yoga's traditional heritage while others actively move away from it and only say the pose names in English. A venue's published content, even the online descriptions of their classes, will give you insight into the persona and character of the venue and how they like their teachers to conduct themselves.

The best research of all, of course, is if you can take a few classes there yourself. Pay careful attention to the teacher's use of sequencing, the difficulty level/general standard of the members, how many spiritual/philosophical elements make their way into the class and other details you pick up on.

You want to stay true to how you teach, of course, but to teach in a variety of places you also need to adapt to the "house style" where needed.

The audition set-up

A yoga audition is typically done in bulk, with 10-20 teachers invited along for assessment and each given 5-10 minutes to teach the room. Occasionally, the audition will be one to one with a studio owner or representative.

Clearly, this is not a natural teaching environment; you are teaching other yoga teachers for one thing, not yoga students or hobbyists. This means the overall standard of practice is likely to be very high, though you will be expected to pretend otherwise during your audition and make verbal/physical adjustments as though it were a typical class. Naturally, the tension in the room is heightened by the unspoken fact that everyone is aware that this is a pass/fail situation leading to a work opportunity.

When you enter the audition, before things get started, try to stay calm and have a chat with your fellow teachers – whether you pass or not this is a great free networking opportunity. For the most part, everyone will be aware that this is a pressured situation and try to ease it out with a laugh and smile; it's pretty rare to encounter dismissive or diva yoga teachers (though occasionally you will).

It's always worth noting that, much like an acting audition, the true audition begins the moment you step into the room and the auditioner may be noting how you engage with your fellow teachers from the start.

Audition sequences

If you've already been covering classes, or even teaching friends, you will know how quickly an hour can fly by. The few minutes you are given in the audition room will be a mere blink in comparison; you have a very small window to show what you can do as a teacher so it's important to make the most of it.

So what should you include? Here are the key ingredients I've found for the ideal audition:

1. **Short sequence:** Select a few key moves which you are confident teaching. Don't try to cram as many postures in as possible and don't worry about repeating the flow on both the right and left sides of the body. Keep it simple!

2. **Tick the boxes:** Use your limited time and sequence selection to show that you can include anatomical adjustments, key visualisations and spiritual elements which make up a well-balanced yoga class. Be sure to show some of your personality and style in

there too.

3. Move and adjust: Be sure to show in the audition that you are comfortable leaving your place at the front of the class and make physical adjustments on students (provided you have made sure they are happy to be adjusted). Just be aware not to turn your back too often as many auditioners do not like this.

Don't 'wing it'

Due to the uncertain nature of auditions, I've spoken to many yoga teachers who prefer to turn up on the day and improvise on-the-fly. For seasoned Vinyasa Flow yoga teachers this is understandably second nature.

But in my experience, this is a terrible idea. In two of my early auditions I outlined roughly in my mind what I would do in terms of sequences, thinking I would fill in the blanks with whatever seemed right in the audition room at the time. I failed both those auditions.

When you turn up on audition day, especially if you are a relatively new teacher, you will be nervous. Just as with regular teaching this is entirely natural and you should certainly not feel ashamed of it, but it does mean that those little asides, jokes and visual descriptions which come entirely naturally when teaching a regular class will not necessarily be there. You will potentially find yourself stumbling over phrases and even unable to bring to mind your go-to teaching scripts.

The solution is to have your script prepared, at least to some degree.

Script it out

After two failed auditions, I was about 70% nerves when going for the next one. I questioned everything at that point: Did I even deserve to be here? Were all the classes I'd taught up until now just due to blind luck? Was I just going to fail again?

Since this audition was for one of London's most popular studio chains, I decided this time my approach had to be different. I resolved to be so prepared that they could not fail me, even if they wished to! I would tick every box possible so that, at the very least, I would be admitted onto the cover list.

I scripted out my chosen sequence, based heavily on the feedback I had received on my previous (not-so-successful) auditions. I then rehearsed it several times so that I knew exactly what I wanted to say in each pose and how to keep the flow moving forward if I stumbled at certain points or lost my way. This also allowed me to include a broad spread of the anatomical, the visual and the spiritual in my script – even pre-planning points when I wanted to demonstrate my use of humour.

Sample Audition Script

Below is a sample of the audition script I used in my successful studio audition. As you can see I used a small selection of moves to roadmap several key aspects of what I think makes my yoga teaching unique. Don't think of the below as an 'audition cheat sheet', but rather a sample of what worked for me. Consider the poses which you really relish reaching and the one-liners which work their way into your classes again and again to build out your own winning audition script. If you're stuck, use your yoga journal to brainstorm your sequence; even mind-mapping it out can be useful.

Top tip: I now actively choose to do my auditions using the 'left' side of the body, as nearly everybody else will do a power flow sequence on the right.

Tadasana/Mountain	A short opening/grounding meditation with the option to talk about 'bandhas'/energy locks of the body and

	add a little spirituality. I also use this brief time with eyes closed to ask anyone in the audition room who would not like moved/adjusted during the sequence to raise their hand. Giving students the option to say "no" to hands-on adjustments is extremely important and will show the auditioner that you have factored this consideration into your flow.
Parsvottanasana/Pyramid (one side only)	Visualisation prompt: "imagine a light from your heart is shining over your front toes." I also used this pose as an opportunity to move and adjust in the audition room too (note: even if nobody actually needs adjusting, showing that you are comfortable with physical adjustments can be a key part of the audition process).
Vrksasana/Tree (one side only)	I use this to demonstrate various arm options, showing that I do not keep my poses static with a "one size fits all" philosophy but allow classes to explore their own variations. Anatomically, Tree is a good pose to give the "extend through the crown/drop down through the tailbone"

	prompt.
Virabhadrasana B/ Warrior 2	Alignment cues are a great way to open this pose, asking the room to bring the front heel in line with the arch of the back foot and drop shoulders from the ears. I also like to prompt the "Drishti"/soft yogic gaze over the middle finger of the extended hand. If there's time to dive deeper I also use this pose as a chance to ask students to balance the fiery strength of the body with the gentleness of the gaze and breath, feeling the sun/moon balanced energies in the body and mind.
Vinyasa	Demonstrating different options for the vinyasa (Chaturanga Dandasana or knees/chest and Cobra/Upward Dog) depending on time.
Adho Mukha Swanasana/ Downward Dog	Another great opportunity for alignment prompts, inviting students to lengthen the spine, open across the shoulders and root down through the heels of the hands. You can also give Child's Pose as a restorative option here and a great way to close your audition sequence.
Seated pose of choice	Personally I like Navasana/

(if there is time)	Boat Pose as it has a lot of variations to offer. I use it as a chance to bring in some humour offering "Jane Fonda-style Pilates pulses" as an extra challenge for the pose before finishing with a gentle forward fold to close.

Less is more

This is definitely a mantra I've found to keep front of mind for auditions and you may have already clocked this, given that the sample script above (the one which resulted in a pass) is only seven poses long. I've noticed that some teachers turn up and try to show off their large vocabulary of postures, squeezing as many as possible into the allotted time. I've also noticed that a certain 'competitive' element can sneak its way into the audition room too, with teachers trying to out-do one another in the intensity, complexity and difficulty of their flows.

There is absolutely no way you can show your full range as a teacher in ten minutes or less. And it's certainly not a case of whoever makes up the hardest sequence 'wins'. So pick postures you are comfortable with and can demonstrate well, along with other elements of the yogic practices which are genuine to your teaching style and gel organically with the language you would normally use in a classroom.

Rehearse

Sadly, unless you have a phenomenal memory, the script will not be in your mind after just writing it out. You need to practice practice practice.

Practice your chosen sequence and script several times before your audition, to the point where you could drop yourself into it at any point and find your way out. As mentioned before, nerves will take over on the day to a greater or lesser degree, so you want to have your audition in both your mind and muscle memory. Forgetting a point or even a pose is common, due to the aforementioned nerves, and you need to be able to pick yourself back up with no-one in the room any the wiser.

I found it useful to have a couple of really key points for each posture; moments where I wanted to make a specific prompt such as "imagine you're squeezing a block between your thighs" or "extend up through the crown as you drop down through the tailbone". Many teachers (myself included) improvise these lines to a greater or lesser degree in a class situation, but always keep in mind the audition room will feel palpably more tense compared to the relatively relaxed atmosphere of most classrooms.

Following the audition you want to have no regrets. If you've put in the time, done the work and give the best effort you can possibly give you will have nothing to reprimand yourself with after.

Rejection part II

Sadly, rejection is a part of the audition process too. It could be that you were not a fit in terms of personality or style, sometimes it's even down to the music you chose or how much eye contact you made (believe it or not, my failed audition feedback has included criticism on both those points). With most venues and chains, you are able to audition again in six months time – so, again, think of it as a "not yet" rather than a "no".

If possible, always ask for feedback from your audition. It can be tough to hear but, in the long-term, this is often where your biggest learning curves will come from. Take note of what they say and when your head is clear (so not directly after), self-analyse it in your yoga journal. Take stock of where you feel you got it right and how you can use any critiques in future auditions.

A not-often talked about truth regarding auditions is that, sometimes, the deck can be stacked against you from the start. The venue may have auditioned you despite having a policy of only hiring teachers with at least two or more years experience; they may have been specifically looking to hire male teachers, female teachers, Ashtanga teachers, Kundalini teachers – the list of possibilities is endless. Despite this, don't take the rejection as a personal attack but simply one of the necessary aspects of walking the path of a yoga teacher.

Try not to beat yourself up, take it all as learning and look to the next opportunity.

It's a two-way street

Auditions can feel like a giant scrum of yoga teachers trying to all get through the same door, but it's worth remembering that the process is there for your benefit, too.

Are you right for this particular venue? Do they appear to truly value their teachers or view them as disposable commodities? Do you get on well with the management or do they turn you off? Are the typical clientele going to be students who will appreciate your teaching? Or are you just chasing a new opportunity for the sake of it?

You don't have to fall in love with every place that you teach, but a good relationship with both the staff and students will make working there a lot more pleasant.

There is one high-end studio which, at the audition, I very much wanted to be a part of: the pay was significantly higher than average and they projected an air of offering top-quality yoga. I was told at my audition that they would happily put me on the cover list but that their clientele (most of whom came from extremely wealthy backgrounds) were very specific about the style of yoga they wanted. Moreover, they would regularly complain to management about teachers they did not like.

Despite the lure of a shiny name on my yoga CV, not to mention more money, I did not pursue this opportunity. I knew that if I were to go through a string of customer complaints it would affect both my confidence and my enjoyment of teaching there.

As you learn more at the audition, trust your instincts and be honest with yourself – if a venue, manager or particular clientele doesn't feel right to you, chances are they aren't.

Remember, you have every right to say 'no, thank you' to an opportunity even if it's offered.

Final word on auditions

After re-thinking my audition technique for that studio chain audition, I was happy to say that I passed.

Not only that, but I was promptly offered two weekly classes mere days after my audition and before I had even had a chance to take any initial cover work. That's not intended as a humblebrag – it brought home to me the power of preparation when it comes to forging your own opportunities and making the audition process work for you.

Auditions may not be the fun part of a yoga teaching career, but learn how to master them and you'll stand head and shoulders above the competition.

Open the door to opportunities, take all you can from mistakes, and you'll be well on your way to a great teaching career.

STEP 6: MARKETING, CONNECTION & COMMUNICATION

So once you start covering classes and auditioning, where does it go from there?

As we've explored, you can use every cover class to open doors to other jobs. This includes more cover, cultivating private clients and turning them into permanent classes on the venue's timetable to name but three. This can be aided by growing your personal network and starting to market yourself both offline and online.

It's important to note that many of these opportunities take time to bear fruit, which is why you want to sow as many seeds as possible. But you'll have to find a certain amount of patience, too. I completely sympathise if you're champing at the bit to get started – patience is not a virtue I'm good at cultivating! But the truth is that after you've made your pitch the decision is largely out of your hands; it rests with the managers, head offices, clients and members.

In some cases, it took several months for a potential private client to decide they wanted to start lessons with me, or a space to open up on a gym's class timetable which I could take over. Use the information outlined in Chapter 4: Attitude, regarding making every cover class count for you and keep in mind the wise words of the Roman philosopher Seneca:

"Luck is what happens when preparation meets opportunity."

Let management know you are looking

When you have the students at a particular venue actively cheer-leading for you, management will usually listen. When you follow up in your emails to management, be sure to let them know that you are open to permanent opportunities on your timetable. If you hear nothing after a few weeks, follow up again.

Keep it polite and of course don't spam the manager's inbox, but if you've proven yourself to be reliant, helpful and popular with the members you want to press yourself forward as much as possible. Nobody gets a prize for being a wallflower, especially in this market.

The same goes for students at the end of class. As I said before, each one is a potential new client, as are all their friends! My own personal sign off is "If you, or anyone you know, is interested in private yoga classes please take one of my cards with you." This can be particularly effective around Christmas time or pre-holidays when people may already be turning their minds to their new fitness and wellness regimes, or ways to gift yoga to loved ones.

The power of reaching out

In my teacher training, we were told that there was very little point in reaching out 'cold' to gyms and studios – basically emailing or calling out of the blue with no prior connection or contacts there.

In many cases, this is sadly true. Popular venues are oversubscribed with wannabe teachers and it helps if, at the very least, you've attended classes there regularly. This is another reason why cover work can be such a powerful foot in the back door, so to speak, as you bypass a lot of the red tape which can constrict the 'official' way in.

Yet if you do feel you would be a good fit for a particular venue, sometimes fortune really does favour the bold. A good example of this in my early teaching career was popular London gym chain Fitness First. A housemate of mine at the time was encouraging me to reach out to the local branch, as she felt sure that my teaching style would gel with them. I was hesitant, given what I'd been warned in teaching training about "cold calling", but with nothing better to do one morning, I gave it a go.

I hit Fitness First up on Facebook Messenger, explaining that I lived very close to this particular branch, had had some success teaching/covering in other London gyms, and would be very interested to know more about the application and audition process. A reply via Messenger promptly informed me that the Group Exercise Manager I needed to speak to was at the gym until midday; she'd been informed I was interested and I was welcome to drop by anytime that morning to speak with her.

Within ten minutes I was walking down the road, certificates in hand and mentally going over the key points I wanted to get across about how I structured classes, what I had learned in my teaching experience so far and what my specialities were as a yoga teacher. One 40-minute in-depth chat later and, having sold my skills well, I was signed onto the cover list. A week later I had my first cover classes at Fitness First and a mere two months down the line I was on the timetable with my very own Wednesday evening Hot Yoga class – the very one I would run off to after informing my digital marketing clients that I was now a proud full-time yogi!

Taking the risk and reaching out may end in nothing more than a terse rejection email (I've had plenty of those to confirm that's true), but that's not to say taking that initiative won't sometimes lead to something wonderful.

Keep growing your network

The best way to find new opportunities is to be on the radar of those in a position to offer them to you directly or who know people that can.

Therefore it's key to keep growing your network of contacts, just as you would if you worked in sales or PR. As you get more ingrained with gyms or studios, some will host socials for their teachers to get to know one another, which can be invaluable networking opportunities. If not, look up yoga, meditation or fitness/wellness/spiritual professionals meet-ups in your area.

This is a great way to meet other teachers, get new ideas and discover fresh opportunities which may never even appear online.

Go local

In my first year as a teacher, I've actually found old-fashioned 'offline' forms of marketing to be far more effective (both in terms of time and money) in terms of growing my business than online ones.

We've already explored one, which is having your business cards handy and encouraging students to take them. But taking advantage of any free local advertising can yield powerful results too. Keep an eye out in local coffee shops or supermarkets for community noticeboards where you can pin your cards or flyers advertising your services.

I've also left my info and business cards with local concierges in luxury apartment complexes, whose residents are likely to be able to afford my services as a yoga teacher, along with doctor's surgeries and hotels.

None of these are guaranteed to yield results of course – I'd argue that no single form of marketing is guaranteed to bring success. But explore every avenue and over time you will reap the results.

Create a 'signature sequence'

As new yoga teachers, it is common for our first flows to mimic, to a greater or lesser degree, the exam sequence from our training. I noticed, even a year after graduating, that while many of the postures and flows may have changed the essential format had remained.

As you break away and move from teaching student into fully-fledged teacher, you will find that some aspects of your training remain and some are replaced with moves, phrases and sequences which feel more right for you. This remixing is a beautiful and highly creative process which is part of what transforms you into a truly unique yoga teacher.

As this naturally happens, developing your own "signature sequence" can become a powerful tool in your teaching. This is the sequence which really represents you and will be comprised of the poses and flows you feel most comfortable teaching. The moves which first come to mind for potential audition sequences can be a useful starting point here.

A signature sequence is an incredible fall-back for a teacher. As fired up as you may feel, especially at the start of your teaching career, there will be days, times and classes when you feel tired; when you are ill or mentally not in your best place. Falling back into your signature, the flow which feels entirely natural for you to guide others through, is an incredible comfort. This is also a great go-to when asked to cover classes at very short notice.

The set of moves which I now think of as my "signature" is also very versatile. For example, I can dwell longer on certain aspects of it in order to apply it to a Power Flow class or I can easily edit or eliminate other sections to apply it to a Gentle Flow/Hatha class.

Your signature flow, just like your own yoga practice, will undoubtedly change and evolve over time. As you discover and grow your vocabulary of both physical postures and verbal phrases (Chapter 8 has more information on sources you can tap into for inspiration on these) and learn to trust in your teaching you will start to sense what you naturally want to keep and what can be discarded.

This is also a great prompt for your yoga journal, as tracking how the flow and sequence which you think of as your 'signature' evolves is a reflection of your growth as a teacher. Sketching or scribbling out the poses which your most enjoy teaching and putting side-by-side is also a great way to initially finding what your signature sequence is. Naturally, if you've already started teaching classes some may have begun to emerge in your scripts.

The discovery and evolution is one of the most magical parts of getting to teach yoga, so stay open and enjoy the journey.

Reliability

Strange as it may seem, I have heard more than one instance of a yoga teacher simply not turning up to a lesson they had been booked for.

Now emergencies happen and are part of life, as do mistakes and the best-laid travel plans. But cultivating an attitude of reliability is paramount to enjoying a long and successful career in teaching yoga. There are many opportunities out there, but don't be under any illusions – it's a smaller industry than you might think it is and people (ie managers) do talk.

Familiarise yourself with the emergency processes and procedures for each gym or studio you are working or covering in and follow them accordingly. For example, some will have a specific duty manager you need to contact in cases of a no-show. Have these procedures and any numbers saved on your phone – you don't want to be scrabbling to look this all up on-the-fly.

Unless the situation is life or death, strive to never leave a venue hanging by simply not showing up. This is highly unprofessional and really scuppers your chances of building a good relationship with them (and as I said, managers talk). Sometimes even doing this once is enough to get your name black-listed or having the class taken away from you as management must then offer compensation to the students for the class.

Part of proving yourself is not just bringing your creativity but your consistency – showing up on time, every time and making yourself a reliable asset.

A word on websites

Do you need a website? The truth is having one is entirely up to you.

I didn't have a website for the first year of my teaching as, honestly, I didn't feel I needed or particularly wanted one. I used Instagram for content strategy but relied primarily on cover work and word-of-mouth recommendations to grow my business.

Having a website is very much meant to be an active part of your online marketing and modern Search Engine Optimisations (SEO – how your site shows up from searches on sites like Google or Bing) is all based around uploading fresh and relevant content.

There are also fees attached to running a website, including the cost of the domain (owning the web address) plus any developer costs if you're not going to build it yourself, which you can now do relatively easily thanks to platforms such as Wix or Square-Space.

Some yoga businesses have been built on the strength of a good website, but it is something else for which time has to be factored in so be aware that it is something which will require ongoing work and attention. If that's not something you want to be bothered with at this point, then relieve yourself of that pressure. Starting with just some social media marketing is fine, which we will explore in the next chapter.

If you're thinking of launching your website, the following is a good idea to gather:

1. High-res images of you. Especially landscape-style pictures to use as banners.

2. Testimonials or positive reviews from classes/private clients.

3. Edited and checked copy which succinctly describes you, your teaching style and why you love to teach yoga (check your yoga journal for ideas!).

Finally, don't be afraid to hustle

There are many ways to communicate and market yourself as a yoga teacher, but remember that you are the owner of your own business and the buck stops with you, so don't be afraid to hustle and sell your services. Jump on seasonal trends, particular groups, underserved markets or any other ways you can think of to bring those new opportunities to you.

While you naturally want to temper this by not being too pushy or in-your-face about it, many yoga teachers suffer from being overly modest and reluctant to sell their services hard; they feel like they should wait at the back until they're called forward and don't want to be imposing. Throw that attitude out right now.

There are ever-evolving opportunities and individuals waiting out there for your services. To get to do what you love, you have to make them aware of you and communicate with confidence that your services are worth paying for.

STEP 7: SOCIAL MEDIA

Previously we explored how to use the cover groups you find on Facebook to land work. But your mind may already have turned to social media and its uses as a personal marketing tool.

This is a very broad topic and there is no way I could cover all the possibilities here, so we'll stick to the most important aspects. Social media can be a powerful asset when it comes to self-promotion, but as you saw with the Facebook Groups, there are rules. Too many people also see social media as a "quick fix" or "fast pass" form of marketing.

Yes, social media has catapulted some yogis into superstardom, but usually that is because those individuals worked for years to build their communities. If having thousands of followers is what you aspire to, you're probably going to be disappointed with the amount of time and effort (and money, in some cases) that it takes to create that.

Plus, word to the wise, having thousands of social media followers may lead to some free swag now and then from Lululemon or Sweaty Betty, but oftentimes it's not the passport to a life of travel and glamour it is sometimes painted as being. Lots of followers may look nice, but can sometimes belie a lack of real substance.

Start with why (again)

Look back at why you want to teach – that's where the substance is. With the channels, tools and choices for social media now being so vast, knowing why you want to teach is a powerful starting point.

Firstly, this will give you an idea of 'who' you want to teach. The temptation is to auto-respond with "everyone", but try and break it down a little deeper to the type of yoga practitioner you feel most comfortable teaching. If you think that you're skewing into a maturer demographic, then platforms such as Facebook or LinkedIn may be where you want to invest your time. If you're thinking younger fitness-aware individuals, you might want to explore Instagram or Snapchat.

As you go back to the why of why you wanted to teach the yogic practices, let this inform the content you might create. Have a think about what online content and the topics it touches on inspires you as you scroll, surf and browse online?

Maybe you like to listen to videos which dive deep into yogic or new age spirituality as you have your morning coffee? Maybe you're inspired by the poses you see on Instagram? Maybe you feel you want to be a voice for change in the world of yoga, and want to do more to promote inclusivity and diversity in classes through insightful blog posts?

Remember that social media channels are not just there to sell classes (that would get really boring really fast). They are there to give an insight into you as a teacher and who you are as an individual. That is what audiences both in and out of the classroom are going to connect with and inspire them to turn up.

Another aspect of the 'why' is to consider why your social media marketing is going to be there. Remember that, unlike using social media for personal connection and creativity, using social for business is there to serve a purpose: to raise the awareness of your brand and, ultimately, get more people interested in parting with money for your lessons. Just like the classes, social media for business isn't for you – it's for them.

Choose your channels carefully

Many people and many brands (and keep in mind I used to work in digital marketing) make the mistake of trying to be on everything. You won't have time.

Choose your channels carefully, based on which demographics you want to go after and why. You're going to have to invest time, so you may as well make sure you enjoy the process as much as possible.

You are much better off doing one channel very well than trying to do everything badly. That doesn't mean you can't develop and explore as you grow, or use content across different channels, but pick the one which best plays to your strengths and your business goals to be your primary channel.

Choose your content

Think about which type of online content you're going to enjoy creating. Do you see yourself as a writer, as a video creator, as a photographer, or as a combination of media?

Go with what feels right for you and don't worry too much about what is statistically going to get you the most likes/followers. As I said before, you want to enjoy the process of creating your marketing content in a way that is genuine for you.

If it's of interest, video is the medium which statistically moves through social media with the greatest ease. The algorithms of Google, Facebook, Instagram and Twitter all favour video above everything else, especially when it is uploaded 'natively' to the platform (rather than posting a YouTube link to Facebook, for example).

If increased reach is your primary goal and you feel comfortable in front of a camera, creating videos of some kind is the way to go.

Remember: it doesn't have to be like everyone else

When I say "videos about yoga", that doesn't necessarily mean flows or physical asana guides. There are loads of those on YouTube with many channels devoted to them. If that is most definitely your area, then you are more than welcome to add your voice to the choir, but with the knowledge that it will be difficult to stand out there.

Sometimes it can be beneficial to try and dive a little deeper into what you can do differently, whether that is a specialisation based around a specific market or diving into an aspect of the yogic practices which are not so commonly explored.

Be true to the parts which you truly find most interesting, not the ones you feel you should be making content about, and you will attract like-minded viewers.

Consistency is king

A popular buzzword in the world of digital and content marketing is "content is king"; I would take this a step further and say "consistency is king".

Look to find consistency with your content, perhaps aiming to put out 1-2 new posts each week, rather than several posts one week and then an elongated radio silence. Just as you can't leave a venue hanging when you have a booking, you can't leave online audiences for weeks without an update. Whether it's written blogs, videos or picture updates, find a schedule which works and is manageable for you.

An option employed by social media managers the world over is to use scheduling software to plan out updates and when you want them to launch. For large-scale social media campaigns on big brands, these are often written and scheduled days or even weeks in advance, even if they look very much in-the-moment. Some platforms you can even use for free, such as Hootsuite and Tweetdeck.

Now that I'm no longer working in the industry I prefer to simply update my social media week-to-week as I like to keep it as authentic as possible, but forward planning is never a bad thing.

Paid social

This is another thin end of a very large wedge, but if you operate any sort of social media for a business you've probably been prompted by options from the social media networks to put money behind, or 'promote' posts.

When you promote a post you can choose who and where you want to target it to. This is particularly useful when you want to increase engagement and views on a particular piece of content. You can also do this with event pages, which is handy if you're organising your own yoga classes in community spaces.

Along with promoted 'posts' you can create advertising campaigns on platforms such as Facebook, Instagram, Twitter or LinkedIn using Ads Manager. These are more complex than just promoting posts but allow you to go into far more detail with how, who and where you want to send your message as you can get extremely specific as you specify the audiences for your ads. As with regular social media content, using media which relies more on picture and video than copy and writing is the surest way to get the most for your marketing dollar as you target your audiences.

If social media and the advertising options which they can bring are something which you see being a key part of your yoga business, check out Social Media Examiner (www.socialmediaexaminer.com) and their weekly podcasts, which can be found on iTunes, Google Play etc.

This site, and all the brilliant info they put out, was my secret weapon when working in the corporate PR world to finding the latest social media tools and trends.

No social? No problem

Just like when it comes to running a website, if social media is truly not your bag then that is OK. Quite honestly it's better to do nothing at all with it than half-heartedly because you feel you 'need' to be on it.

As stated before, and speaking as someone who worked for several years in the world of PR and digital, it's always worth remembering that beyond all the online and offline ads, content, web pages, influencers and everything else, the most powerful form of marketing is still word of mouth.

The biggest takeaway is this: social media and online content only work when it's genuine. And in this digital-savvy world, it's very easy to spot online media that is clearly there just to be there and not because it serves any real purpose. So if the idea of having a Facebook page to promote your business or vlogging your thoughts into your phone camera fills you with dread, just remember that it's by no means essential.

Besides, letting that myriad of online marketing options take over your brain is one of the leading contributors to what we will explore next: Getting burnt out with it all.

STEP 8: BURNOUT

As a new, or relatively new, player in the yoga teaching game it may be hard to imagine getting burned out. I remember being on such a high after my first teaching experiences I just wanted to do it again and again!

Enthusiasm is a wonderful elixir to empowering yourself and forging ahead when it comes to that all-important creative thinking around new opportunities.

But once your business starts to grow and your timetable fills, whether that's in a full or part-time teaching capacity, it can be easy to find yourself just moving from class to class without a great deal of thought or consideration. This, I've found, is an early stage of burnout.

We should always strive to give a lot to our classes. At the end of the day, people have paid to be there and you need to give them value for their coin. But giving so much of yourself is draining on both the body and the mind, to say nothing of the spirit.

Any entrepreneur can also relate to the deep and all-consuming obsession which can creep in when trying to take a new business off the ground.

What does burnout look like?

Symptoms of burnout include:

- Feeling robotic: You lurch from appointment to appointment like an automated teaching machine. You may even start to realise you are simply teaching the same sequence over and over on repeat.

- Guilt: You start to feel guilty for daring to take time away to do anything else other than your yoga business.
- Exhaustion: Physical and mental tiredness, with a lot of lethargic "can't be bothered" feelings.
- Lack of concentration: You find yourself starting to procrastinate and putting off the tasks surrounding your teaching, such as admin and preparation.
- No control: Feeling like the schedule and timetable are controlling you, not the other way around.
- No satisfaction: No matter what you achieve or do it never feels like enough.
- Happiness 'when': You lose enjoyment with what you are doing or achieving at present and continually find that your inner monologue is putting happiness out of your reach; telling you you'll be satisfied when you reach the next goal, payment level or stage of teaching (truth: you won't).
- Physical symptoms: Headaches, migraines, unexplained aches and pains or cold/flu-like symptoms.
- Less sleep: Either because you are burning the candle at both ends, or because when you do try and sleep your mind replays endless round of your to-do lists!
- Loathing: Sometimes, when more than one of the above start to come forward, you can even find yourself hating what you once loved.

Burnout can be hard to avoid because starting your own business so often begins as a labour of love. And it's a labour which is never finished. There are always going to be more emails to send, marketing avenues to pursue, techniques to master and new business opportunities to explore. Your to-do list can easily become bottomless if you let it.

Burnout can manifest in many ways, but after six months of taking my yoga business full time, it manifested for me as physical illness. I felt myself starting to get sick, but I covered it up with painkillers and carried on. The result? I completely lost my voice and became so ill I was forced to take a whole week off. My body literally forced me to stop.

As the physical practice of yoga is living proof of, our bodies are strong and capable of incredible things. But they're fragile too and if you don't give yourself down-time to recover your physical self will find ways to make you.

Find your strengths

A great way to manage burnout is to hone in on your strengths – where in your teaching career are you strongest? This could be a style of yoga that really energises you, it could be treasured local classes vs those you have to travel further to get to, or it could be public vs private (more on this in the next chapter).

I know that my strength is in public classes. As a former per-former, I adore the thrill of holding a large room and drawing them into the narrative of the class. I enjoy private classes and clients a lot too, but I find them harder. The preparation, for me, is much deeper and in the private setting I feel obligated to bring much more energy into the room; contrasted with public classes where I feel like I receive a lot of energy back from a group of 20-30 students.

This is my personal preference and I know yoga teachers who would say the exact opposite. They love the intimacy of teaching one to one or in small groups and find big public classes draining or frustrating, given that you are constantly looking for the safe median or middle-ground between what you want to teach and what is possible, where there could be a vast difference in terms of fitness level, strength and flexibility.

As you teach more and explore different classes, styles and ways of interpreting the yogic practices, start to ask yourself where you really think your personal strengths lie as a teacher. Be totally honest here and try not to simply hone in on the opportunities which will make you the most money – they may well be different.

The classes you feel strongest and most empowered to teach are, long-term, what you want to try and fill your timetable with.

Learn your limits

So in terms of avoiding burnout, this means that I know I can teach around 3-4 public classes a day maximum (including travel time etc) but probably only 1-2 privates.

After that, my own energy starts to lag and I feel myself going into "going through the motions" mode. My philosophy is that when you're being paid to be there, whether in a public or a private capacity, just going through the motions isn't fair on the students or on yourself. You have to give it more than that.

I also find admin a huge drain on my energy – the big invoice push at the end of the month is a task only to be tackled with coffee and chocolate close to hand. Even throughout the month, the aforementioned bottomless pit of spreadsheets, emails, personal marketing, follow-ups, to-do lists and everything else can easily start to feel overwhelming. Part of accepting my own limits is accepting what I can do and prioritising accordingly and that, sometimes, that it's OK to zone out and watch a movie without the laptop open on my knees.

Learning your own limits can be a tough lesson – sometimes we have to take it beyond in order to know what and where the limit is. But this is something that you will sense into the more you teach, especially if you are taking this business full-time. Knowing your limits does not make you weak; it helps keep you jogging along at a steady pace rather than sprinting for a short stint and then crashing out.

Chasing a new opportunity or more money is, let's be honest, a tempting prospect. But as I frequently tell yoga students: It all starts with respecting your body and respect your mind.

Without them on-side you won't get far.

Balance it out

As with so much of life, balance is the key. Know what you can do, accept what you can't do so much of, and design your timetable accordingly.

As with any job, we have to acknowledge that there are going to be aspects of it we don't love or even opportunities we take for the money more than the joy and job satisfaction it brings. That is part of creating a business, taking the opportunities that you can find and being your own boss.

Sometimes, of course, we are our own worst judges when it comes to analysing how much or how little we can do. The yoga journal can be an invaluable tool here, but sometimes it can be even more helpful to turn to our support network: our loved ones. My family and close friends now know to tell me when I've taken on too much and when I am slipping back into the trap of not allowing myself any time off.

Again, it may sound mad to a new yoga teacher, but sometimes it can be much harder to allow ourselves time off than to keep working ourselves raw.

Take time away

Giving yourself down-time is key to avoiding burnout. You will find that running your own business can quickly come to dominate any free time you have and, as mentioned, this can sometimes come with a deep sense of guilt when you try to let it go along with an obsession to take it ever-further.

There are going to be days when you don't want to do any yoga (yes, I'm very aware that #yogaeverydamnday is an Instagram thing). This also means days when you don't want to study spiritual texts, work on your flows, or even do business admin. This is not only OK but essential and necessary!

Take time out to explore other things you enjoy and remember that, while yoga may be your career or a part of your career, it is not your whole life. Even those who work intense hours during the week in a 'regular' job get some down-time at the weekend (anyone I've found who claims to work all day every day is usually exaggerating to some degree, or winds up having a complete physical breakdown). Your brain needs time to reset.

And to keep your teaching fresh, sometimes you need to take a step away from it and remember there are other things which also enhance and enrich your life.

Key takeaways

In this mad modern world where everything has to be done faster, bigger, better and more flawlessly than yesterday, burnout is a very serious and real epidemic. How strange and ironic to think that scientists and philosophers at the turn of the century predicted that, by this point in human evolution, we would not be working at all!

As a yoga teacher and yoga entrepreneur, it may be that you feel you need to keep working to justify yourself. Early in 2019 when I took yoga full-time, I had more than one person refer to my new career and business as a 'hobby' and asking if I was going to get a 'real job' again. One of the fallouts from this was I felt I had to work non-stop and earn as much money as possible to justify it. An attitude that I still content with.

But working until you are at the point of exhaustion or to heighten your perceived image in the eyes of others isn't going to lead you anywhere good, and certainly not in the direction of a long and satisfying yoga teaching career.

STEP 9: DEDICATION AND STAYING INSPIRED

So once you've got your first taste of teaching and are starting to get an idea of your own personal strengths and weaknesses, where do you want to take it?

We touched on this in Chapter 8 – you'll likely already have found that you discover more about teaching the more you do it. And before long, your individual preferences will start to emerge.

Maybe you prefer teaching those one to ones over classes? Perhaps, like me, leading those big groups from the front gives you a thrill like nothing else? What about when it comes to style? It could be Power Yoga fires you up, or that you prefer the cooling energies of Yin?

As you gain more experience, pay attention to the styles and classes that you truly relish and look forward to preparing and teaching. Keep making note of them in your yoga journal. As always, be honest and contrast them to the ones that start to feel more workaday or that you really are doing just for the cash (again that's not necessarily a bad thing, but just be aware of it). Most teachers start out as generalists, but as you climb the yoga teaching ladder many studios like if you have a specialisation.

Look back again at those reasons you first outlined for wanting to teach. Perhaps they've stayed the same or perhaps, as you start to build your yoga teaching experience, they look radically different? Either one is OK.

Delving into the depths of why you wanted to teach, what you're teaching now and where you want to take it in the future, is a powerful way to both keep yourself grounded and avoid stagnation with your teaching career. In between the busy moments of teaching, marketing and admin, taking time to reflect and consider is a great way to be clear about where you want to take your talents – along with giving yourself a bit of self-care.

Inspiration

Along with taking time away to give your mind a break from teaching yoga, it's important to keep yourself inspired. When you're un-inspired, this is when you usually find yourself moving from class to class teaching more or less the same set of moves over and over. And that gets pretty boring pretty fast.

Sources of Inspiration 1: Other classes

The single best way that I've found to re-inspire yourself as a yoga teacher is to attend other teacher's classes. They will inevitably do things differently to you and, even if you don't love the lesson, I guarantee it will give you ideas for new sequences, variations on classic poses, fresh themes, alternative styles and other ideas.

Going along to a yoga class is also a way to remind yourself of what it feels like to be a student again. I sometimes get so caught up with trying to give the best lessons I can that I forget! This is particularly true when it comes to beginners: remember how intimidating it was when you first took the plunge to go to a yoga class? No matter how strong and dynamic your flows get you still want to keep the class open and make that first experience of yoga magical.

Going back to class and letting yourself be a student again is a great way to get inspired for future teaching.

Sources of Inspiration 2: Online teachers

Checking out teachers online is another great way to get new ideas. I try to watch a couple of different online classes a week, across different styles, to fill my mind with new moves, phrases and flows. Some of these I may lift directly, others I will adapt to my own style and my own classes.

Feeding the mind with lots of new ideas without overloading it is the best way to find that inspiration and keep bringing new ideas to your classes, not to mention that watching teachers online is a great resource that you can tap into almost anytime.

Note: Getting inspired does not mean directly copying the whole thing. Nobody owns the yoga poses or any variations thereof, but it's unlikely that lifting an entire sequence or script would work. Allow yourself to take the elements which feel right for you, that resonate with your inner teacher, and discard the rest.

A few of my personal recommendations for YouTubers are:

Cat Meefan	Especially useful for Power Flow/ Dynamic practice styles, Cat is brilliant at coming up with new takes on classic Vinyasa yoga guaranteed to challenge even advanced yogis. This includes new Vinyasa Flow ideas, along with options for really powering up your practice and working into areas like shoulders, arms and abs.
Yoga with Adriene	YouTube's favourite yogini, I find Adriene's philosophy of creating flows for all ages and practice levels a fantastic source of inspiration, particularly when planning out gentle and beginner-

	friendly classes or sequences for private clients who are newer to yoga.
The Honest Guys	My personal favourite meditation channel on YouTube, The Honest Guys are second-to-none when it comes to creating guided meditations. I regularly use this channel both for my personal meditation practice and for inspiration when it comes to writing meditation scripts, particularly for corporate clients. Everything from tone to timing and conception to content is a meditation masterclass, whether it's a quick morning mindfulness guide or a cinematic guided meditation set in Middle Earth.
Yoga with Kassandra	Kassandra's videos and explanations on Yin were a massive source of inspiration when I began delving deeper into this style. If you're looking to add Yin elements to your practice, wondering how it differs from standard yoga classes or want ideas for Yin sequences then Kassandra's channel is the place to go.
Brett Larkin Yoga	Another great resource for bringing it back down when you need to design something more beginner-friendly, Brett interspaces her themed asana videos with info on yogic spiritual practices, alignment cues and meditations.
Man Flow Yoga	If you're looking for physical forms of asana practice with a complete lack of bandhas, chakras etc. then this channel is a great place to start. Between

	the flow videos you'll also find tips on motivation, dedication and what to do about gnarly pain spots in the body. Now personally I always think the spiritual elements are what make yoga yoga, but if you're looking to design a more fitness-based flow then these videos are invaluable.
Five Parks Yoga with Erin Sampson	Along with a dynamic creativity which will inspire (and re-inspire) your sequencing, Five Parks Yoga videos are filmed around Costa Rica and Colorado, meaning you also get to enjoy some gorgeous vistas along with great flows.

Sources of Inspiration 3: Anything you like!

I always find it both fascinating and magical that, when it comes to feeding that creative side of ourselves, inspiration really can strike anywhere. And sometimes, stepping outside of the world of yoga to get inspired can be incredibly liberating.

Maybe running or dancing or finding new ways to move your body will give you fresh ideas of what to bring to the mat. Perhaps long walks in nature or observing animals will feed your mind.

I've been inspired by anything and everything from nature documentaries to films to theatre shows; when it comes to getting inspired there are no rules. This is another great use and benefit to keeping a yoga journal. When inspiration strikes, get it down on paper whether it's in the form of a written entry, sketch, mindmap or doodle so that you can develop and dive into it later.

You never know, even the yoga journal itself could become a source of inspiration as you add more to the pages and re-interpret past ideas.

Further study: the spiritual

Most yoga courses contain at least some introductions into the history and philosophy which has shaped yoga into the modern practice that it is today. My advice is to carry that study forward. Dive deeper into the sacred texts and sutras which you began studying on the course and keep reading them. Remember that with books on the sacred and spiritual there is rarely a 'right' or 'wrong' way to interpret them (much like our bodies and minds interpreting the poses on the yoga mat), so use this study time like meditation – you're simply going to stay open and see what arises in your interpretation of the text.

I enjoy expanding this study beyond yoga. This includes aspects of religion and history which are other branches on the same tree, such as Hinduism, Buddhism and Taoism, along with New Age and other 'modern' re-interpretations of ancient spiritual practices.

This isn't about 'converting' or subscribing to any particular spiritual dogma, it's about expanding the mind and awareness by looking at how others have interpreted some of the secrets and mysteries of our world and the universe beyond. Whether it's nature paganism, prescribed religious rituals or just working with individual energy, throughout the ages we have found many windows to interpret the infinite – peering through someone else's window without judgement is a great way to expand your own thinking.

While reading spiritual texts for yourself can be time-consuming (if very rewarding) remember that our modern digital world is still exploring the same dichotomies that we have been for aeons. Podcasts or YouTube videos are great to tune into and give yourself a hit of spiritual study on the go.

Further study: the anatomical

While pondering the etherial mysteries of the universe, it's also good to remember that yoga is also a celebration of the physical body and all its marvellous capabilities. The anatomy that we study in teacher training is, again, a mere hint at what lies beneath or the surface of our skin and diving deeper into how human bodies are put together can only enhance your teaching.

As you deep-dive into our shared human anatomy, this is also a great way to start theming classes or creating workshops around different body parts which often hold lots of stress and tension, such as hips, core, hamstrings or shoulders.

Podcast recommendations

I find podcasts an invaluable resource as they are perfect for listening to on-the-go. This means that even when bombing around London on the trains and tubes (which I spend a significant amount of most days now doing) I can still be increasing my learning and feeding my mind.

This actually comes back to something that I did as a student on my yoga teacher training – with very little home-time to revise due to freelance workloads, I recorded my notes as audio tracks which I could listen to as I travelled.

Below are some of my favourite podcasts to subscribe to, but don't be afraid to search out the ones which are going to engage you and spark that magic interest of learning. Inspiration is entirely individual and exploring what feeds our own minds is part of the joy. But as a starter when it comes to learning more about yoga why not try:

Yoga Talks	J. Brown dives deep into many aspects of yoga, from business to history to teachers of the past, present and future. J isn't afraid to ask the questions you might be thinking and provides

	a meaty learning experience with every episode.
Yoga Land	Former Yoga Journal alumna Andrea Ferretti explores many facets of the yogic practices, from asana to Ayurveda. You never know what is coming next with this podcast, whether it's exploring different styles of yoga, teacher self-care, anatomy or tips for your wellness business.
TriYoga Talks	In-depth interviews with some of Triyoga's international roster of teachers. This is a great way to deep-dive into some of the individual philosophies and stories of the teachers themselves, many of whom are fantastic individual characters with many years of experience under their belts.
Elevated Elephant	Host Rachel Perry was my own course leader at Yoga London and her podcast is filled with her signature warmth and enthusiasm for all aspects of the yoga practice, from choosing music to how to organise retreats, with some fantastically knowledgable guest stars.
The Connected Yoga Teacher	Much more than a podcast full of business gems, the tie-in Facebook Group and other online resources have created a thriving online community to help support you as you navigate the challenges of growing your yoga business.

And when it comes to stepping outside conversations directly about yoga, I highly recommend:

Happy Place	Fearne Cotton's podcast asks some of the big questions around physical and mental wellbeing with some of the biggest names in British media. A bit lighter in tone than some of the others if you want some feel-good and empowering easy listening.
Under The Skin	Russell Brand talks to international stars of stage, screen and self-care. Brand's signature charm and wit keep the episodes entertaining throughout and he's another host who's not afraid to ask the hard questions you might be thinking.
Deliciously Ella	Especially good if you want to add a bit of knowledge around food and nutrition to your repertoire as a teacher. Ella also tackles what to put in our minds as well as our stomachs to stay healthy.
Star Wars Theory	OK, this is usually just when I want to nerd out on Star Wars lore a bit. But the links between the Jedi and yogic philosophy run deeper than you might think (another secret source of geeky inspiration).

Final word on staying inspired

Although it often comes from outside sources, like new information and learnings, we have to ultimately take responsibility for our own inspiration as yoga teachers.

This means you have to take the initiative yourself; giving yourself time to explore, create and attend. This very much relates back to also avoiding the burnout and making time for ourselves (with the caveat that, some days, having no yoga in your life is OK!).

New ideas are your life-blood as a yoga teacher and you need to find time to seek out that inspiration. Without it, you will quickly find yourself descending into stagnation and falling back onto the same teaching script. While this may not be immediately noticeable to students, it can quickly become dull to teach and your lack of motivation will become very clear very quickly.

Getting to teach yoga is a tremendous gift and, as a teacher, never forget that you hold the power to serve as an inspiration yourself – or if that sounds a bit too lofty remember that you hold the potential power to simply make someone's day a little better. I regularly think back to how important yoga classes were for my own mental and physical wellbeing, especially when going through darker periods of life, and try to always remember any student could be going through something similar.

Serve your students first and foremost by bringing new ideas, new scripts and new movement variations into the classes, to challenge both their minds and bodies, along with your own!

STEP 10: FAQS

Outlined below I've tried to cover some of the big questions which may still be lingering in your mind. While I've tried to make this guide as comprehensive and concise as possible, there is no way to cover everything. These last questions are a combination of my own, or the ones I remember having while still sitting in my bedroom with that teaching certificate in my hand and many, many queries in my head, along with some ideas from other yoga teachers I've spoken to.

If I've not been able to answer your question, either here or throughout this manual, my contact details can be found at the end of the book. You're welcome to drop me a line via email or Instagram and ask me!

I'm extremely nervous about teaching my first class, what can I do?

Honestly, and I understand it may not be the answer you want to hear, but you just have to jump in. In fact, the sooner the better. Because the longer you put it off the more pressure you will put yourself under. Accept those jittery feelings (we all get them) but tell yourself that you are in control of the nerves; they do not control you.

Put in the prep before you teach your first class and decide on a flow which is going to be simple and enjoyable for you to teach. The first class will be over before you know it and you'll see it wasn't nearly as frightening as you made it out to be in your head.

Then you'll be on a roll.

My personal practice isn't very advanced, can I still teach?

When I first went into my yoga teacher training I couldn't do a headstand. Looking back, I probably also had a lot of work to do on my core strength and alignment, too.

The truth is that most of the attendees to your classes will be beginners or, at most, intermediate. Only a tiny percentage of classes are targeted towards advanced yoga practitioners as most gyms and studios want to attract as many people as possible.

You can still put a strong and dynamic yoga class together without advanced postures. And there's nothing that says you have to demonstrate them, even if you do include them. Just give the option for anyone who "has them in their practice" and leave it at that. In many cases now I actively choose *not* to demonstrate advanced postures. This is because, in a group class setting, I do not want those who are not confident in their practice trying them and potentially injuring themselves.

Keep in mind too that physical asana is only one part of the yoga practice and is only a conduit to connecting the mind and body to prepare for meditation. There are many other facets you can bring into your classes beyond more difficult poses.

I'm teaching my first private client and they can barely do any of the poses, what do I do?

First of all, and as we've explored, one of the hardest things as a new teacher is letting go of your exam sequence. Remember that, to a new practitioner of yoga, this is likely going to be very hard indeed! Secondly, keep in mind that in teacher training you have been working with other aspiring yoga teachers, who will be operating at a very different level of practice to your average new yoga student.

If after your first lesson with the new private client it's clear that most of the common or 'classic' yoga poses are too much for them, break it down and make it simpler. Get creative with what you can do in tabletop pose, letting the student keep more contact with the floor. From standing, try different variations of breathing and twisting. Perhaps slowly build up their strength and flexibility until they are moving through a whole sun salute unaided, modifying the practice as much as you need for their capabilities.

Tailor each and every lesson to their body and their mind and what they can do to progress, and to feel that progress. Just because they do not have the skills yet for classic yoga does not mean they cannot learn to move mindfully and with awareness.

Sometimes these are the most satisfying of all clients to teach and watch grow.

I'm terrible at memorising sequences and keep mixing up my left and right, what can I do?

There's a secret that I have for this: Choose moves which can be done on both sides of the body.

For example, if I bring a class into High Lunge as part of a Vinyasa Flow sequence I'll get them to twist to both the right *and* the left on each side. That way, no matter which order I do the twists in, I can't miss one out!

Also, if you have trouble memorising sequences just keep them super short. Do a couple of postures on each side (right/left), either separated by a Vinyasa or a reset standing at the top of the mat. Lots of teachers aspire to long, choreographed sequences but I always found these rather dull and difficult to follow, which isn't really what I want when I go to class.

How do I make the leap from part-time to full-time teacher?

This is a big one. The best advice is to plan, plan, plan. Don't just take the leap and assume the universe will fall into place for you. The hard truth is that it just doesn't work like that and trusting to blind luck is never a good idea. In fact, it's often a one-way track to ending up disappointed.

Be honest with yourself and ask if devoting your full-time work to teaching yoga is truly what you want, both in terms of job satisfaction and income. If it is, look at where you need to take your current teaching roster to make that leap. How much do you have to earn for the books to balance? How many more classes or clients will you have to take on in your week? Do you currently have the contacts to make those opportunities happen or is that time which will have to be factored in?

Give yourself time to plan it out before you take the plunge and accept from the start that any form of self-employment, at least initially, is usually a lot more working hours than a regular 9-5. The 'payoff' is that the satisfaction with what we do is significantly higher.

Sometimes it is also a question of savings – do you have enough saved up to be able to pay the essentials if you have a "lean month" when it comes to earning money from teaching yoga? Any business, and hence any business owner, will have fluctuations month to month (especially at the beginning) and need a bit of capital in order to get started and launch the business.

Many yoga teachers think of money and finances as a dirty topic and are reluctant to discuss them. But in any business, the finances dictate almost everything and to quote more wise words from my Dad: "Failing to prepare is preparing to fail."

I just did my first class and everybody

looked really blank and bored! Does that mean I'm a terrible teacher?

The face that we make when we are deep in concentration or focus is usually much the same as the one we make when bored (ironic, isn't it?). There is every chance the students were simply deep in their practice, which of course is exactly where you want them to be!

Frankly, even if they were bored that is not your problem and not a reflection of your teaching. You're not there to be a performing monkey or keep classes entertained throughout; you are there to create a safe space for moving meditation. If some students choose not to go to that place then that is something they need to work on in their own practice.

As we've covered, some students are not going to gel with you and, just occasionally, some will choose to show this on their face – or even tell you after that you are not teaching it the same as the regular/previous teacher.

The only thing you can do is accept that you are not going to be everyone's cup of yogi tea and move on. As, hopefully, will they.

How much "woo-woo" is too much?

OK so behind the scenes I know a lot of yoga teachers who are seriously into the woo-woo (a broad term covering all aspects of spirituality, mysticism, New Age philosophy and the 'alternative'). I loved attending classes where teachers would flavour the flows or themes with a unique personal touch – such as handing out 'Intention Cards' before the class to provide a personal touchstone for the practise or inviting students to write down any dedications/affirmations for the energy of the class before it begins.

Other teachers like to include elements of traditional yogic philosophy, such as bandhas, koshas or chakras, while I've known others to open the practice with chanting, quotes from Buddhist/

Hindu/Taoist philosophical texts, excerpts from poems, plus "energy cleansing" or other rituals.

Again, these are beautiful ways with which to individualise your class and personalise the teaching space.

However, the deeper down the road into the alternative that you go, the more you have to accept that this is going to turn some people off. Some students want to come to yoga purely from a fitness perspective; others may be entirely new and get scared that they are being indoctrinated into some sort of New Age cult. Some gyms or studios may even have opinions on this and how much it should be a part of the class, especially as pertains to aspects of religious symbology.

As I mentioned, my personal opinion is that the spiritual aspects are what make yoga yoga, as opposed to Pilates or HIIT. But if you're unsure, keep it neutral. Asking students to set an intention for the class or take a moment of gratitude at the end for their body and mind can sometimes be enough.

The most important thing is to keep it genuine to you – don't try to copy anyone else simply because you feel you have to in order to be a "real yoga teacher".

How do I stop myself talking
too much in class?

If you tried to say everything there was about a pose in terms of anatomy, alignment, visualisation and spiritual connotations you wouldn't get through more than three poses per class.

But sometimes editing ourselves as teachers can be a challenging part of honing our skills. Try to limit yourself to a couple of pointers per posture. I try to really look around the classroom for these and take in a general sense of what is going to be most useful to that particular group. If there are lots of rounded backs, prompt lengthening the spine; if a few students are clearly collapsing into the back knee in Warrior 1, give a verbal adjustment for that. Along with verbal adjustments you want to give the students the silence and space to be in their own practice too.

A couple of regular students are asking for more challenges, but this class also attracts a lot of beginners. How do I keep them happy and strike the right balance?

The art of teaching classes, especially large ones, is finding that middle-line which is going to please, and challenge, as many attendees as possible.

Some students truly do feel, however, that the class is not complete without an advanced set of inversions. A good window for this is right before savasana. As you bring everyone into relaxation, invite the class to take "any final movements, twists or postures to complete their practice". Those who feel the need will take some time standing on their head or balancing on their hands, while those who don't will already have their eyes closed and so not feel pressured to mimic.

If you are getting a lot of pressure from a small student minority over this, explain to them that the class contains beginners to yoga and kindly ask that they respect this – advanced asana is best done in a small workshop environment under the watchful gaze of a specialist.

Most importantly, do not let yourself feel pressured into teaching anything that you do not feel comfortable with. Very often, to be frank, I've found that this request primarily comes from students who are looking for an excuse to indulge their ego and show off in a public setting.

I'm not a pregnancy teacher, so

what do I do if someone pregnant shows up to my class?

Firstly check your insurance and how it is worded. Depending on the type of insurance you have, and at what stage of pregnancy the student is at, you may not be insured to teach them at all. In this instance, you would have no choice but to explain this to the student and politely ask them not to attend the class (better dealing with the fallout from this after class than an emergency during).

Personally, I've had a few instances of heavily pregnant ladies turning up to open-level gym or studio yoga classes.

When they have informed me at the start of the class, I first ask whether they are already familiar with yoga (most are – if they are not, I would advise against them doing the class). Yet even if they are familiar with the practice, and especially if the class is labelled "Power Flow", "Dynamic Vinyasa" or similar, I explain that they are welcome to stay but should modify as they need – not going deep into twists etc.

It would be unfair to the other students to radically change the flow on account of one person, especially if they have turned up expecting a strong physical challenge. You need to stick with what has been presented on the venue's timetable. If necessary, inform the student that she might consider seeking out specialist yoga classes in pre- or post-natal yoga, which would be done under the safe supervision of an expert. It is also worth checking an individual gym or studio's policy on this.

Ultimately, a student's body and mind is their own responsibility during practice. As neither a doctor not a therapist, you can only guide and inform.

How do I stop people using phones in class?

This is an absolute no. It is distracting, not just for you as the teacher, but runs the risk of spoiling the class for fellow students.

If someone is using the 'rest time' in Downward Dog/Child's Pose to text or scroll, I would stop by their mat and politely ask them to turn off their phone during class. If this is a running theme week-to-week make it part of your pre-class checks. I'd even spin it as a positive: Ask everyone to turn off all mobile phones and un-plug from the outside world for a bit; invite them to ground and be present in their practice.

FINAL WORD

Well, there you have it.

I've passed on all I can tell you after one year of teaching yoga myself and it is my sincerest wish that this guide helps and informs you to start your yoga teaching career, in whatever form that manifests.

Remember always that, just like the practice of yoga, the journey of a teacher is never truly finished. That is the profound beauty of teaching – the more you help others to learn, the more you will discover you yourself want to keep learning, in an infinite spiral of knowledge which never stops.

As you may already have gathered, the history of yoga is a convoluted one. While it may be marketed as an ancient or esoteric practice by modern studios, from what I can gather we do not truly know in what form it first began. Likely that it did not even begin as a physical practice at all, but one of chanting and meditation. From that it could even be theorised that yoga, in some form or other, has always been with us; even long before we put a name to it.

Yet however tenuous the link between our modern practice and how ancient yogis first conceived it, the techniques and traditions in all their myriad forms have made their way down through the millennia, one way or another, interpreted and re-interpreted, to come to us today. It's a humbling thought, but while you honour that history take the teaching and pass it on in the way that instinctively feels right for you.

If your teaching instincts don't feel that well-honed yet don't worry; keep going and, over the months, you will find your own voice start to emerge from the choir.

Here's a final truth to take away with you: The writing of this guide, just like how I fell into my yoga teacher training, happened almost by accident. I was gunning for a guest spot lecturing on business at a yoga teacher training course and, sadly, I was not successful. But the knowledge and ideas which had formulated in my head for my proposal refused to lie dormant and I resolved to write them down. If you are reading this now I do still wish, in many ways, I could have workshopped it all out with you; heard your feedback and opinions and answered your questions.

But once I started writing the flood did not stop and I can only hope, humbly and sincerely, that these words have helped or even inspired you in some way as a yoga teacher. And if you are still writing in your yoga journal I hope that your own words will inspire you more.

For me, yoga and the teaching of it not only pulled me back from the brink and made me realise there was more to this world than the grind and graft of the corporate world and all the expectations which go with it, but it gave me a deeper appreciation for the mind and body we are blessed with along with a resolve to do the most with them that I can.

In the words of American humorist Erma Bombeck:

When I stand before God at the end of my life, I would hope that I would not have a single bit of talent left, and could say, 'I used everything you gave me'.

Go forth, dearest yogi, and use everything that you have. And if you have questions or feedback, I will do my best to answer them at markbonington@gmail.com or you can contact me via Instagram @markbonington.

If you are in London, I hope to see you on the mat sometime.

With love and blessings,
Mark Bonington

ABOUT THE AUTHOR

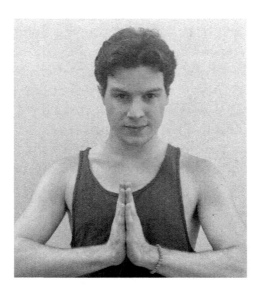

Hailing from Scotland, Mark Bonington currently lives and works in London. Following a career in PR and digital marketing he now runs his own yoga and meditation business full-time.

Mark teaches public classes at MoreYoga, Fitness First and Virgin Active branches across London, alongside working with private clients.

When not teaching yoga, Mark loves writing, running and embracing the cultural side of the capital!

You can find out more about Mark, including how to book private and one to one sessions, at www.markboningtonyoga.com.

Printed in Great Britain
by Amazon

10388690R00058